The Natural No-Heartburn Cookbook

Karin Cadwell, Ph.D., R.N.

Foreword by Steven R. Peikin, M.D.
Professor of Medicine and Head of Gastroenterology
Robert Wood Johnson Medical School at Camden

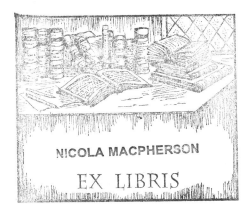

NICOLA MACPHERSON

EX LIBRIS

Sterling Publishing Co., Inc.   New York

For Chuck, who even after 30 years together makes every day full of love.

Acknowledgments

Without the support of my friends and family, who serve as taste testers and critics, I would not have been able to produce these recipes. Many thanks especially to Joanne and Ruth McIlhenny, who have been unfailing in their support, and to Fran McIlhenny, whose specialty is dessert taster.

Special thanks to my daughter Anna, who lovingly contributed time and talent to this project, and to my husband, Chuck, whose dedication to accurate analysis turns the recipes into real tools for a healthier life.

Thanks too to my editor, Hannah Steinmetz, for her wit, skill, and thoughtfulness.

Any errors and omissions are my own.

Library of Congress Cataloging-in-Publication Data

Cadwell, Karin.
    The natural no-heartburn cookbook / Karin Cadwell.
       p.   cm.
    Includes index.
    ISBN 0-8069-5970-3
    1. Heartburn—Diet therapy—Recipes. I. Title.
RC815.7.C33 1996
616.3'320654—dc20   96-13609
                                      CIP

10 9 8 7 6 5 4 3 2 1

Published by Sterling Publishing Company, Inc.
387 Park Avenue South, New York, N.Y. 10016
© 1996 by Karin Cadwell
Distributed in Canada by Sterling Publishing
c/o Canadian Manda Group, One Atlantic Avenue, Suite 105
Toronto, Ontario, Canada M6K 3E7
Distributed in Great Britain and Europe by Cassell PLC
Wellington House, 125 Strand, London WC2R 0BB, England
Distributed in Australia by Capricorn Link (Australia) Pty Ltd.
P.O. Box 6651, Baulkham Hills, Business Centre, NSW 2153, Australia
Manufactured in the United States of America

Sterling ISBN 0-8069-5970-3

CONTENTS

FOREWORD

Y OU WAKE UP in the middle of the night with a burning feeling beneath your breastbone. Sitting up seems to help, but you continue to suffer until you scour the medicine cabinet for a bottle of your favorite antacid. The discomfort resolves after several minutes, but two hours later the same thing happens again.

You're at work. You bend over to tie your shoes and the next thing you know, you have a sour taste in your mouth or, worse yet, some partially digested food from the lunch you ate an hour ago.

You develop a feeling of pressure beneath your breastbone and even though you occasionally have heartburn you wonder, "Is this a heart attack?"

Does this sound like you? Well, you're not alone. Forty-four million adult Americans suffer from gastroesophageal reflux disease, otherwise known as GERD. GERD is a constellation of symptoms including heartburn, regurgitation, chest pain, and difficulty swallowing. It's also a structural disease of the esophagus, including esophagitis, esophageal ulceration, peptic stricture (narrowing of the esophagus), and Barrett's esophagus. According to a Gallup poll taken a few years back, seven percent of Americans experience heartburn on a daily basis and 25 percent have heartburn at least twice a month, making it one of the most common problems that brings a patient to the doctor. Even people with asthma, chronic cough, and hoarseness may have GERD contributing to these problems.

A simple trip to the pharmacy or grocery store proves how common heartburn is. You can see row after row of heartburn remedies, including antacids, which come in all different shapes and formulations: calcium, magnesium, aluminum, or alginic acid–containing antacids. You can find over-the-counter H_2 blockers, such as Pepcid AC, Tagamet HB, and Zantac 75. Visit your doctor and you are likely to get a prescription for H_2 blockers or, in difficult cases, proton pump inhibitors such as Prilosec or Prevacid. In all, the U.S. market for heartburn remedies is well over a billion dollars in sales per year.

While many people with significant heartburn symptoms require prescription medication at some point in their lives, the majority have mild, intermittent symptoms and may never require drugs. The Gallup poll I previously referred to determined that most people with heartburn never consult a doctor, preferring to treat themselves. Most of them know that the best way to treat heartburn is with diet. While diet doesn't seem to help ulcer disease of the stomach or the duodenum very much, it is an extremely important part of the treatment of GERD. Many people skip dietary therapy in favor of strong drugs that suppress acid secretion or that tighten the valve at the end of the esophagus. These people end up taking medication indefinitely, some of them not realizing that there is a natural remedy every bit as important as taking medication.

Dietary therapy of GERD really works. Some foods that we eat can relax a valve at the end of the esophagus, permitting stomach acid to go back up into it, causing symptoms and damage. Avoiding those foods may be all some people need do to control their heartburn. Additionally, most of the foods we need to avoid are not necessarily very healthy for us (e.g., fat), so other health benefits may result from a diet to treat heartburn. People with heartburn who don't try dietary therapy before going on prescription diets may be wasting money and subjecting their bodies to lifelong medication they might not even need.

Most physicians recommend treating heartburn in a stepwise fashion. The initial step always includes elevating the head of the bed on six-inch (15 cm) blocks so that gravity returns refluxed acid back into the stomach. It also includes the dietary therapy well outlined in Dr. Cadwell's *The Natural No-Heartburn Cookbook*. This book should help most readers eliminate or at least reduce their symptoms of heartburn and may help them avoid taking medication. Readers will soon discover that avoiding heartburn-producing foods doesn't mean a bland, monotonous diet. The recipes in *The Natural No-Heartburn Cookbook* are very appealing and tasty and should become an important part of your heartburn treatment.

Steven R. Peikin, M.D.
Professor of Medicine
Head of Gastroenterology and Liver Diseases
Cooper Hospital/University Medical School
Robert Wood Johnson Medical School at Camden, New Jersey
author, *Gastrointestinal Health*

Chapter 1

INTRODUCTION

IDEAS ABOUT HEARTBURN and acid stomach problems have changed. The old approach was to lower the amount of stomach acid by drinking large quantities of milk and cream and sticking to bland products, such as baby food. But researchers found that although this did cut down on acid for a while, the rebound of acid production was high.

Nowadays, doctors and researchers understand that the problem is more than just the amount of acid in the stomach. In fact, in most people heartburn and a burning, full feeling in the chest are probably symptoms of GERD, or Gastro Esophageal Reflux Disease (often just referred to as "reflux") This unpleasant sensation tends to occur if a one-way valve positioned between the esophagus and the stomach becomes a two-way valve. This valve, called the Lower Esophageal Sphincter (or LES), normally works by letting food and liquid into the stomach and then preventing food from traveling back the other way up the esophagus. A lower esophageal sphincter that is weak (or "relaxed") allows the strong acids from the stomach to flow back up into the tender esophagus. The acid then comes into contact with the esophageal lining, which results in the symptoms known as heartburn.

Some factors associated with this problem have nothing to do with food. Tight clothes can increase pressure and make stomach contents push through the LES into the esophagus. So can straining to have a bowel movement or straining to lift something heavy, which can contract your abdominal muscles and push up against the LES, opening it the wrong way.

Lying down after meals can also cause heartburn in people with a weak LES. So, avoiding a supine position for about three hours after meals can help prevent reflux. Also, many people who can't get relief during the night have found that sleeping leaning up against a pile of plllows or putting the legs that support the head of the bed up on 6 or 8-inch cinder blocks can help ease the discomfort they feel. This keeps the flow downward, into the stomach, and away from the esophagus. Not eating within three or four hours of bedtime is also a good idea.

Some prescription medications for other gastrointestinal complaints, asthma, high blood pressure, or angina may have the side effect of relaxing the LES and causing heartburn as a result. Talk to the doctor about the side effects to find out if any other prescription medication options are available. Of course, sometimes a specific heart, high blood pressure or other drug is so important, it will be necessary to do other things (such as follow a no-heartburn diet and sleep on an elevated bed) to reduce the likelihood of heartburn.

Of course, over-the-counter antacids are widely used to counteract the burning sensation of heartburn. They come in several varieties, often with aluminum or calcium as the active ingredient. You may be one of the many people who have been using antacids for some time and feel that you are just too dependent on them. Maybe you are worried about taking in too much aluminum or calcium. Maybe you are tired of the yo-yo symptoms caused from the rebound of lowering the amount of stomach acid with over-the-counter antacid preparations and then experiencing even more heartburn when your stomach responds normally by producing even more acid.

Maybe you would like to try to cut down on the expense of over-the-counter or prescription drugs that relieve your heartburn symptoms. Maybe you just don't like being so dependent on these ways of dealing with heartburn and would like a more natural approach to good health. This cookbook can be a great second step. The first step is to have an honest chat with your health care provider. Make sure your symptoms really are heartburn and not something else. When you are sure, try the easy, healthy, and delicious recipes in this book.

The Essentials of the No-Heartburn Diet

Lower Fat
Fat stays in the stomach longer than other foods and has a tendency to relax the LES, so heartburn may result.

The recipes in this book are not fat-free, and a fat-free diet is not the goal here. Fat is an important part of a complete diet, in proportion to other foods, of course. Fat coats the nerves, for example and is vital to the body's functioning. The trouble is, most of us tend to have too high a percentage of fat in the diet on a daily basis.

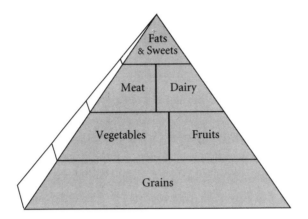

The food pyramid puts fats in the following proportion:

You can easily see that the food pyramid gives the smallest space to fats. That is what each of us needs to do every day. By now, nearly everyone knows that olive oil and canola oil are preferred over palm oil, coconut oil, cottonseed oil, and "vegetable oil." But the butter *vs.* margarine choice isn't so easy. In recent years, experts have gone back and forth about butter and margarine. I'll leave the choice to you and your personal health care provider, but as far as health is concerned, whichever you choose, use it sparingly.

Get in the habit of reading labels. Watch out for prepared foods that boost the amount of sugar so the percentage of calories from fat is lowered. Look for the *number of grams* of fat per serving. Most people should get around 30 grams of fat a day. Ask your health care provider if that's okay for you.

Eating the recommended amount of fat is a low-fat diet for many of us. I've worked hard to get the most taste for the lowest amount of fat in the recipes in this book, but eating a Danish during your coffee break (16 grams) or spreading cream cheese on a bagel (10 grams) can negate your careful cooking, so be watchful of added fats.

I have used skim milk in the recipes for your low-heartburn diet and I also call for many fat-free products that are now available at the supermarket. Eaten alone, most cannot be considered yummy, but in a recipe with enough other flavor, they work just fine. These nonfat foods put recipes back into a heartburn-decreasing diet that would have been off-limits a few years ago. Try the cheesecake, for example. You won't believe how good it is.

Smaller Portion Size

Overeating at any one time can cause heartburn and acid stomach. Going without is not the answer either. Try to not skip meals or eat too fast. Don't eat within three hours of going to bed.

Some people are much more comfortable dividing their total daily calories into five or six smaller meals. The trick here is to avoid adding two or three additional meals. If you do that, you'll just be overeating more often, and that won't help your symptoms! The portion sizes in this book are fairly standard. That means they are smaller than you might expect—more like those of airplane meals than the generous portions you might expect at your favorite restaurant.

Higher Fiber

Fiber helps all kinds of gastrointestinal (G-I) problems and can be a real help to people with acid problems. For example, increased fiber plus increased fluids makes stools softer, bulkier, and easier to pass with less straining. That means less backward pressure on your LES and a decreased chance of reflux and heartburn.

Of course, a higher fiber diet has many benefits beyond helping with heartburn and other G-I complaints. Eating more fiber helps you feel more satisfied, especially on a lower fat diet, and can help with weight loss. Being overweight all by itself can put pressure on the LES and cause heartburn. Losing weight can make a difference. Lower fat and higher fiber is an essential component of healthy weight loss plans.

Sometimes, higher fiber diets might not be advised for people with a specific problem, such as diverticulitis. If your health care provider has told you to stay away from higher fiber, continue to do so. But check. Many physicians are finding that higher fiber diets are great for problems they used to think required low fiber diets.

Fiber is thought to be important to maintain blood sugar levels, cholesterol, and blood fats and prevent heart disease and cancer. So there are good reasons to increase the fiber in your diet.

There's more to fiber than bran. Oats, beans, seeds, nuts, whole grains, fruits and vegetables are loaded with fiber. You'll find these ingredients all through the recipes in this book.

Lower Spiciness

Some spices can stimulate acid secretion and add to the problems of a weak or relaxed LES. Often the problem seems to be more than the spice itself. It's the spice in conjunction with too much high-fat food. A person experiencing reflux and heartburn can almost taste or sense the spice. Often the spice gets blamed. After an enormous Italian meal at a restaurant with bread and butter, a few glasses of wine, and huge servings of a main course, you may get heartburn. The portion sizes, alcohol, and fat don't get the blame. Garlic does. You may say, "I really can't eat garlic. It gives me heartburn." That's because you can taste and sense the garlic and not the fatty overeating that's very easy to indulge in at a wonderful restaurant.

Yes, some spices can stimulate increased acid production. To find out which ones bother you, keep a food diary. Write down what you eat, how much, and if you experienced heartburn within three hours or so after eating. See which spices bother you.

According to Dr. Steven Peikin, author of *Gastrointestinal Health,* the spices most often linked to stomach symptoms are:
- Black pepper
- Chili pepper
- Mustard seed
- Cloves
- Nutmeg

You won't find them in recipes in this book except as optional additions. The recipes taste just fine without the optional items, but

may lack what has come to be the traditional flavors. Dr. Peikin also points out that:
- Garlic
- Chili powder, and
- Curry powder

can be irritating for some people. There are no recipes that call for chili powder or curry powder in this book and if garlic bothers you, just leave it out. Garlic is not essential to any recipe.

Spices and herbs such as cinnamon, allspice, mace, thyme, sage, paprika, caraway seed, rosemary, and basil are usually not a problem. But these, too, should be considered optional for you if they give you trouble. Try experimenting by substituting flavors that you like and that don't bother you.

Acid-Producing Foods and Beverages

Orange juice, grapefruit juice, and tomato juice bother most people who suffer from acid stomach, reflux, and heartburn. These juices can be especially troublesome on an empty stomach. If you love orange juice but it bothers you, try squeezing it yourself. Fresh orange juice may cause you less heartburn than pasteurized or concentrated varieties. Again, try not to drink it on an empty stomach. Tomato-based foods such as spaghetti sauce and soups with a tomato base are notorious for causing heartburn.

Radishes are another well known cause of heartburn, but there aren't too many people who so long for radishes that they can't give them up.

Peppermint relaxes the LES, so stay away from mint-flavored things, even mint-flavored gums and candies if you have problems with acid. Also, coffee, tea, alcohol, cigarettes, and chocolate can contribute to heartburn. If chocolate bothers you, replace the cocoa powder in recipes with carob powder, which is available at larger supermarkets and health food stores. The problem with chocolate may be the fat that comes with it, so I've put in some reduced-fat chocolate dishes for chocolate lovers to try. Of course if it's not the fat or the amount of food you ate before the chocolate, it could just be the chocolate itself and it may be best to avoid it altogether.

Why is it worth cooking in a new way?
There are no over-the-counter drugs that will cure the burning pain of heartburn. The best you can hope for is symptomatic relief. Prescription drugs may help, but they are expensive and have their own side effects. And some people just prefer a more natural pathway to good health.

Lower fat, higher fiber, lower calorie, less spicy cooking is a healthful way to make an impact on your own life. Try these delicious low-fat, low-calorie, easy-to-make recipes. Many of the recipes are higher in fiber and all have been spice-adjusted. I hope you enjoy them.

Chapter 2
BREAKFAST

B & B Breakfast Smoothie

Blueberries and banana are the two "B's." When it's not fresh blueberry season, use frozen.

1 C	nonfat yogurt	250 mL
1	large ripe banana, cut into pieces	1
1½ C	nonfat milk	375 mL
1 C	blueberries, fresh or frozen	250 mL

Combine the ingredients in a blender or food processor. Mix until smooth.

Yield: 4 servings

Each serving contains:
**calories: 110 total fat: 0.6 g saturated fat: 0.2 g cholesterol: 3 mg
sodium: 93 mg carbohydrates: 20.6 g dietary fiber: 1.7 g**

Blueberry Breakfast Cake

This is a treat on a weekend morning. It's easy to make and smells wonderful while baking.

2 C	flour	500 mL
1 C	sugar	250 mL
3 t	baking powder	15 mL
¼ C	butter or margarine	60 mL
¼ C	nonfat cream cheese	60 mL
2	eggs beaten, or equivalent egg substitute	2

1 C	nonfat milk	250 mL
1 t	vanilla extract	5 mL
1½ C	fresh or frozen blueberries	375 mL

In a large mixing bowl, sift together the flour, sugar, and baking powder. Using two knives or a pastry cutter, cut in the margarine and cream cheese. In another bowl combine the egg, milk, and vanilla. Sprinkle a few teaspoons of the flour mixture over the blueberries and coat the blueberries before mixing them into the flour mixture in a large mixing bowl. Add the egg and flour mixture and combine gently just until it is evenly moist. Fold gently into a 9 x 5 x 3 inch (22 x 12 x 7 cm) lasagna pan that has been coated with a nonstick cooking spray. Bake in a 350°F (180°C) oven for 50-60 minutes.

Yield: 18 squares

Each square contains:
**calories: 139 total fat: 3.3 g saturated fat: 1.8 g cholesterol: 31 mg
sodium: 116 mg carbohydrates: 24.6 g dietary fiber: 0.3 g**

Bagel and Cream Cheese

The old favorite, bagel and cream cheese, is not a problem for most people if they substitute fat-free cream cheese.

1	bagel	1
1 oz.	fat-free cream cheese	28 g
1 T	fruit-only jelly or jam	15 mL

Slice the bagel in half and toast the halves until golden brown. Spread with fat-free cream cheese and jam or jelly.

Yield: 2 half-bagel servings

Each half-bagel serving contains:
**calories: 134.3 total fat: 0.6 g saturated fat: 0.1 g cholesterol: 3 mg
sodium: 261 mg carbohydrates: 26.4 g dietary fiber: 0.9 g**

Easy Breakfast Surprise

A toaster oven is ideal for making this quick and delicious breakfast.

1 slice	whole wheat bread	1 slice
1 t	butter or margarine	5 mL
1 T	cranberry sauce	15 mL
¼ C	ripe banana, cut into coins	60 mL
1 t	brown sugar	5 mL
sprinkle	cinnamon	sprinkle

Broil the bread lightly on one side. On the untoasted side, spread the butter, then the cranberry sauce. Arrange the banana over the cranberry sauce. In a small bowl, combine the brown sugar and cinnamon. Sprinkle the brown sugar mixture over the banana coins. Broil for 30 seconds to 1 minute, until hot and bubbly.

Yield: 1 serving

Each serving contains:

**calories: 220 total fat: 4.9 g saturated fat: 2.7 g cholesterol: 10 mg
sodium: 51 mg carbohydrates: 110 g dietary fiber: 17.1 g**

Granola

Granola has become a popular breakfast cereal. But commercial granolas are loaded with fat. This granola recipe, on the other hand, is surprisingly low in fat.

3 C	oatmeal (regular)	750 mL
½ C	wheat germ	125 mL
⅔ C	sliced almonds or other nuts (optional)	170 mL
1 T	safflower oil	15 mL
¼ C	honey	60 mL
2 T	molasses	30 mL
¼ C	apple juice	60 mL

Mix the oatmeal, wheat germ, and almonds in a flat lasagna or jelly roll pan. In a saucepan combine and heat the oil, honey, molasses, and apple juice. Drizzle over the oatmeal mixture, using a spatula to push the mixture around in the pan. Bake in 325°F (160°C) oven for about 30 minutes. Then, mix again and bake 10 minutes. (The longer you cook it, the crunchier it gets.)

Yield: 9 servings (½ cup, or 125 mL, each)

Each serving contains:
calories: 177 total fat: 3.7 g saturated fat: 0.2 g cholesterol: 0 mg sodium: 276 mg carbohydrates: 31.9 g dietary fiber: 5.5 g

Applesaucey Oatmeal

If cinnamon is a problem for you, just leave it out of the recipe. For a sweeter breakfast, add a little brown sugar.

½ C	instant oatmeal	125 mL
1 C	water	250 mL
¼ C	applesauce	60 mL
½ C	nonfat milk (optional)	125 mL
sprinkle	cinnamon (optional)	sprinkle

Cook the oatmeal in the water on top of the stove or in the microwave according to the package directions. Let it stand for a few minutes before topping with the applesauce, milk, and cinnamon, if desired.

Yield: 1 serving

Each serving contains:
calories: 198 total fat: 2.6 g saturated fat: 0 g cholesterol: 0 mg sodium: 418 mg carbohydrates: 38.6 g dietary fiber: 5.2 g

Oatmeal with Raisins

The secret of this oatmeal recipe is to let the mixture sit for a few minutes. The raisins become plump, soft, and flavorful.

½ C	oatmeal	125 mL
1 C	water	250 mL
¼ C	raisins	60 mL
¼ C	nonfat milk, optional	60 mL

Cook the oatmeal in water on the stove or in the microwave according to package directions. Stir in the raisins, cover, and let the mixture sit for a few minutes. Top with milk, if desired, before serving.

Yield: 1 serving

Each serving contains:

**calories: 258 total fat: 2.6 g saturated fat: 0.1 g cholesterol: 0 mg
sodium: 421 mg carbohydrates: 54.6 g dietary fiber: 5.9 g**

Pancake Batter

Making pancakes from the following recipe takes about one minute longer than commercial pancake mix.

¾ C	skim milk	190 mL
1½ T	safflower oil	22 mL
1	egg or equivalent egg substitute	1
2 t	baking powder	10 mL
3 T	sugar	45 mL
1 C	flour	250 mL

In a large bowl, combine the milk, oil, and egg or egg substitute. Stir in the baking powder, sugar, and flour. Mix just enough to moisten the flour; do not overmix. (The batter should have small lumps.) Preheat a lightly oiled griddle or frying pan *while mixing the batter.* The griddle must be hot; drops of water will sizzle and "dance" when dropped on it. Pour about ¼ cup (60 mL) or less for each pancake onto the griddle or frying pan. With a spatula turn the pancakes when they are bubbly and the edges are cooked. Serve hot. To freeze, cool and wrap the pancakes in freezer wrap. Reheat in a toaster-oven, or microwave.

Yield: makes 16 small pancakes

Each pancake contains:
**calories: 58 total fat: 1.7 g saturated fat: 0.2 g cholesterol: 13 mg
sodium: 55 mg carbohydrates: 9.0 g dietary fiber: 0 g**

Cornmeal Buttermilk Pancakes

An old-fashioned recipe that's worth bringing back. Thin with a little nonfat milk if the batter gets too thick.

1⅓ C	cornmeal	330 mL
¼ C	white flour	60 mL
½ t	baking soda	3 mL
2	eggs or equivalent egg substitute	2
2 C	fat-free buttermilk	500 mL
¼ C	melted butter or margarine	60 mL

Combine the cornmeal, flour, and baking soda in a mixing bowl. In another mixing bowl beat together the eggs and buttermilk. Stir the cornmeal mixture into the eggs and buttermilk gently. Do not over-beat. Stir in the melted butter. Fry pancakes ¼ cup (60 mL) at a time on a hot, nonstick griddle or frying pan. (When the pan is ready drops of water will "dance" on the hot surface.) Turn the pancakes over when the tops are bubbly and the bottoms are lightly brown.

Yield: 12 pancakes

Each pancake contains:
**calories: 126 total fat: 4.9 g saturated fat: 2.7 g cholesterol: 46 mg
sodium: 101 mg carbohydrates: 16.2 g dietary fiber: 1.1 g**

Corn Cakes

You'll be delighted with the taste of these pancakes.

¾ C	yellow cornmeal	190 mL
½ C	(white) flour	125 mL
½ C	whole wheat flour	125 mL
1 t	baking powder	5 mL
2 T	sugar	30 mL
1¼ C	skim milk	310 mL
¼ C	nonfat yogurt	60 mL
2 T	olive oil	30 mL
4	egg whites, whipped until stiff	4

Mix together the cornmeal, flours, baking powder, and sugar in a medium bowl. In a small bowl, mix together the milk, yogurt and oil. Pour the wet ingredients over the dry ones. Mix until just blended. Fold in the whipped egg whites. Heat a heavy-bottomed frying pan coated with nonstick cooking spray. Drop the batter ¼ cup (60 mL) at a time onto the hot frying pan. Fry until the bottom of the corn cake is brown and the bubbles are even on top. Flip the cakes over to brown the other side.

Yield: 12 corn cakes

Each corn cake contains:

**calories: 112 total fat: 2.6 g saturated fat: 0.4 g cholesterol: 1 mg
sodium: 66 mg carbohydrates: 18.2 g dietary fiber: 1.3 g**

New Hampshire Pancake Topping

This topping is especially good on any of the pancakes with cornmeal.

1 C	nonfat yogurt	250 mL
⅓ C	maple syrup	80 mL

Stir the yogurt and syrup together. Serve cold allowing each person to put a spoonful or two over each pancake.

Yield: 1⅓ C (330 mL), or 5½ servings

Each ¼-cup serving contains:
calories: 401 total fat: 0.6 g saturated fat: 0.3 g cholesterol: 4 mg
sodium: 183 mg carbohydrates: 88 g dietary fiber: 0 g

Rice Griddle Cakes

A super way to use up that leftover rice.

1½ C	cooked rice, cold	375 mL
2	eggs or equivalent, lightly beaten	2
2 C	nonfat milk	500 mL
1 T	sugar	15 mL
2 C	flour	500 mL
2 t	baking powder	10 mL

Mix the rice, eggs, and milk together in a medium mixing bowl. In another bowl, mix together the sugar, flour, and baking powder. Add the dry ingredients to the wet ones and mix just enough to moisten. Heat a frying pan coated with nonstick cooking spray. Drop onto the heated frying pan and cook until bubbles form on the surface. Flip the griddle cake and brown on the other side.

Yield: 20 cakes

Each cake contains:
calories: 84 total fat: 0.7 g saturated fat: 0.2 g cholesterol: 22 mg
sodium: 56 mg carbohydrates 15.8 g dietary fiber: 0.1 g

French Toast

French toast is as quick to make in the morning as regular toast and the extra protein from the egg makes it a more balanced food than plain toast.

½ C	egg, beaten, or equivalent egg substitute	125 mL
½ C	nonfat milk	125 mL
¼ t	vanilla extract	2 mL
6 slices	soft whole wheat bread	6 slices

In a shallow bowl mix together the egg, milk, and vanilla. Spray a frying pan with nonstick spray. Dip each piece of bread in the egg mixture, turning to coat both sides. Fry in a heated pan, browning on both sides. Serve hot. Top with maple syrup or a cinnamon and sugar mixture.

Yield: 6 slices

Each slice contains:
**calories: 102 total fat: 3.0 g saturated fat: 0.6 g cholesterol: 36 mg
sodium: 36 mg carbohydrates: 12.3 g dietary fiber: 1.0 g**

Sour Cream Waffles

Keep waffles tender by not overmixing the dough.

1 C	flour, sifted before being measured	250 mL
1½ t	baking powder	8 mL
1 t	sugar	5 mL
1 t	baking soda	5 mL
3	egg yolks	3
2 C	nonfat sour cream	500 mL
3	egg whites	3

Sift the flour, baking powder, sugar, and baking soda into a large mixing bowl. In another mixing bowl, beat the egg yolks until light, with an electric mixer. Beat in the sour cream. Pour the sour cream mixture over the dry ingredients and stir a few times to combine. In a clean mixing bowl, beat the egg whites until stiff. Fold the egg whites into the batter. Spoon onto a preheated waffle iron. Cook until steam stops (about four minutes).

Yield: 4 waffles

Each waffle contains:
calories: 256 total fat: 4.2 g saturated fat: 1.2 g cholesterol: 159 mg sodium: 598 mg carbohydrates: 38 g dietary fiber: 0 g

Eggs Scrambled with Cream Cheese

Without fat-free cream cheese, this recipe would be off-limits to anyone on a low-acid diet. It's still creamy and delicious—almost sinful.

1 (3 oz. pkg.)	fat-free cream cheese	85 g
1 C	nonfat milk	250 mL
½ t	salt	3 mL
	eggs, or equivalent egg substitute,	
6	lightly beaten	6

In the top of a double boiler over boiling water, or in a heavy saucepan, carefully melt the cream cheese. In another saucepan, scald but don't boil the milk. Stir the milk into the cream cheese and add the salt. Add the eggs and cook a minute or more, stirring gently with a fork.

Yield: 6 servings

Each serving contains:
calories: 101 total fat: 5.1 g saturated fat: 1.6 g cholesterol: 216 mg sodium: 329 mg carbohydrates: 3.6 g dietary fiber: 0 g

Egg in Toast Ring

This recipe works well in either a toaster-oven or conventional oven.

1	slice, whole wheat bread	1
1	egg or equivalent egg substitute	1
pinch	salt (optional)	pinch

Use a biscuit cutter to cut the center from the slice of bread. Spray the bread ring with nonstick cooking spray on one side and grill in a frying pan to toast on one side. Line a baking pan with foil and spray with nonstick cooking spray for easy clean-up. Put the toasted side down on the pan. Put the egg in the cut-out center. Bake in a preheated 350°F (180°C) oven for 15-20 minutes, until the egg is set.

Yield: 1 serving

Each serving contains:

calories: 139 total fat: 6.0 g saturated fat: 1.6 g cholesterol: 213 mg sodium: 63 mg carbohydrates: 11.6 g dietary fiber: 1.0 g

Breakfast Banana Bread

Make this bread on the weekend and enjoy it plain or toasted all week long.

½ C	butter or margarine	125 mL
½ C	fat-free sour cream	125 mL
1 C	brown sugar, packed	250 mL
6	eggs, or equivalent egg substitute	6
2 C	flour	500 mL
2 t	baking powder	10 mL
3	bananas, ripe, mashed	3
1 t	vanilla extract	5 mL

In a medium bowl, beat the butter until light and fluffy. Mix in the sour cream and brown sugar. With the mixer on low speed, add the eggs one at a time. In another bowl, mix together the flour and baking powder. Slowly add this dry mixture to the butter and egg mixture. Beat well. Stir in the bananas and vanilla extract. Pour the batter into a loaf pan that has been coated with a nonstick cooking spray. Bake in a preheated 350°F (180°C) oven for 90 minutes. A toothpick inserted into the center should come out clean when the bread is done. Cool for 15 minutes or so in the pan before turning out onto a wire rack to cool completely.

Yield: 16 slices

Each slice contains:
**calories: 194 total fat: 7.8 g saturated fat: 4.2 g cholesterol: 96 mg
sodium: 137 mg carbohydrates: 26.9 g dietary fiber: 0.5 g**

Chapter 3
SOUPS

Cream of Pumpkin Soup

A rich and hearty soup adapted from a traditional New England recipe.

2 T	butter or margarine	30 mL
1 C	onion, chopped	250 mL
2 (10¾ oz.) cans	low-fat chicken broth	2 (340 mL) cans
1 (16 oz.) can	pumpkin	1 (500 mL) can
dash	salt (optional)	dash
3T	sugar	45 mL
¼ t	cinnamon (optional)	2 mL
⅛ t	ginger (optional)	1 mL
1 C	evaporated skim milk	250 mL
¼ C	fat-free sour cream(optional)	60 mL

Melt the butter in a large (2 quart or 2 liter) saucepan or Dutch oven. Add the onion and sauté until tender. Add one can of broth. Stir and bring to a boil. Cover, reduce heat, and simmer for 15 minutes.

Transfer this onion-and-broth mixture to a food processor or blender and blend until smooth. Add the remaining ingredients except the evaporated milk and sour cream. Bring to a boil, stirring well. Reduce heat, cover, and simmer for 10 minutes. Stir in the evaporated milk and heat thoroughly. Garnish each serving with a dollop of sour cream, if desired.

Yield: 6 servings (makes 6 cups or 1.5 L)

Each serving contains:
**calories: 122.2 total fat: 4.0 g saturated fat: 2.5 g cholesterol: 12 mg
sodium: 304 mg carbohydrates: 17.6 g dietary fiber: 1.8 g**

Cream of Mushroom Soup

This is as good as any restaurant mushroom soup and it's not hard to make.

1 t	butter or margarine	5 mL
1 lb.	fresh mushrooms, washed, towel-dried, and sliced	450 g
1 t	lemon juice	2 mL
1 C	water	250 mL
1 t	tarragon	5 mL
½ t	chervil	2 mL
pinch	white pepper	pinch
1½ C	beef broth	375 mL
3 T	flour	45 mL
2 T	fat-free sour cream	30 mL
1 C	skim milk	250 mL
2 T	sherry, or sherry flavoring	30 mL

Melt the butter in a saucepan. Add the mushrooms, lemon juice, water, tarragon, chervil, pepper, and beef broth. Bring to a boil. Reduce heat and simmer for 10 minutes. In a bowl, mix together the flour and sour cream. Add the milk gradually, stirring until smooth. Mix a few spoonfuls of the hot mushroom mixture into the milk mixture. Then mix all of the milk mixture into the hot mushroom mixture. Cook over low heat, stirring constantly until the soup thickens. Stir in sherry. Serve right away, or reheat carefully.

Yield: 6 servings

Each serving contains:
  **calories: 83 total fat: 1.8 g saturated fat: 0.7 g cholesterol: 3 mg
    sodium: 428 mg carbohydrates: 9.9 g dietary fiber: 1.0 g**

Shrimp Bisque

A very economical way to serve shrimp. Speed things up by warming the milk while sautéing the onion.

1½ lb.	shrimp, cooked, peeled and deveined	675 g
3 T	butter or margarine	45 mL
2 T	onion, grated	30 mL
3 C	warm nonfat milk	750 mL
1 C	nonfat milk	250 mL
2 T	cornstarch	30 mL
3 T	sherry (optional)	45 mL
2 T	parsley, chopped	30 mL

Chop the shrimp and set aside. In a saucepan, melt the butter, add the onion and sauté until the onion is soft but not brown. Add the shrimp and the three cups (750 mL) of warm milk. In a small bowl, mix the 1 cup (250 mL) of milk with the cornstarch. Stir into the soup. Heat to the boiling point, stirring constantly until the soup thickens. Add sherry, if desired, and the parsley.

Yield: 5 cups

Each one-cup serving contains:
**calories: 286 total fat: 9.5 g saturated fat: 4.9 g cholesterol: 229 mg
sodium: 387 mg carbohydrates: 13.9 g dietary fiber: 0.1 g**

Corn Chowder

It's the long cooking and browning of the onion that adds the flavor.
Double the recipe if you want more than three servings.

1 T	butter or margarine	15 mL
1	medium onion, finely chopped	1
2	medium potatoes, cut into cubes	2
2 C	skim milk	500 mL
10 oz.	frozen corn*	300 g
⅛ t	fresh pepper	1 mL

In a skillet melt the margarine over medium heat. Cook the onion until the pieces are *browned*. Mix onions, potato cubes, and milk in a saucepan. Simmer over low-to-medium heat for 20 minutes, but do not boil. Add the corn and pepper. Simmer for another 5 minutes.

Yield: 3 servings (makes 2¾ cups (690 mL)

Each serving contains:
calories: 242 total fat: 4.9 g saturated fat: 2.7 g cholesterol: 13 mg
sodium: 313 mg carbohydrates: 43 g dietary fiber: 4.1 g

* If you like thicker corn chowder, substitute a can of cream-style corn.

Creamed Pea Soup

This is a great soup for folks who work or anyone pressed for time.

10 oz.	frozen peas, thawed	284 g
2	cubes, chicken bouillon	2
1	onion, thinly sliced	1
4 T	flour	60 mL
3 C	nonfat milk	750 mL
dash	mace (optional)	dash

Place all the ingredients in a blender or food processor. Cover and blend on high speed until smooth. Transfer to a saucepan. Cook over low heat, stirring constantly until thoroughly heated. Serve warm.

Yield: 6 servings

Each serving contains:
  **calories: 108   total fat: 0.6 g   saturated fat: 0.2 g   cholesterol: 2 mg
    sodium: 541 mg   carbohydrates: 2.7 g   dietary fiber: 7.7 g**

Cream of Celery Soup

Try this soup for Sunday night supper with a sandwich or fresh bread.

1 T	butter or margarine	15 mL
1 C	celery, chopped (including the leaves)	250 mL
⅓ C	onion, chopped (optional)	80 mL
2 C	low-fat chicken broth	500 mL
2 C	nonfat milk	500 mL
2 T	cornstarch	30 mL
2 T	parsley, chopped	30 mL

Melt the butter in a large saucepan. Add the celery and onion, if desired. Add the chicken broth and cook for 10 minutes. Pour ½ C (125 mL) of the milk into a small bowl. Add the cornstarch, and stir to dissolve. Stir this milk mixture gradually into the soup saucepan.

Add the remainder of the milk. Bring to a boil. Cook and stir for 1 minute. Ladle the soup into bowls and sprinkle the top with parsley.

Yield: 4 servings

Each serving contains:
**calories: 101 total fat: 3.2 g saturated fat: 1.9 g cholesterol: 10 mg
sodium: 270 mg carbohydrates: 12.2 g dietary fiber: 0.7 g**

Vegetable Soup

This soup recipe is old-fashioned but a cinch to make. Just throw almost everything in the pot. You'll be happy with the results.

6 C	low-fat beef broth, from bouillon cubes	1.5 L
2	medium onions, peeled and thinly sliced	2
2	carrots, peeled and thinly sliced	2
4	stalks of celery, diced	4
1	small turnip, peeled and finely diced	1
18	string beans, cut into pieces	18
2	potatoes, peeled and cut into small pieces	2
1 C	macaroni pasta (broken, if large type)	250 mL

Put the beef broth in a large pot. Add everything except the pasta and cook until the vegetables are almost tender, ½ hour or so. Add the macaroni and cook 15 minutes more.

Yield: 6 servings

Each serving contains:
**calories: 220 total fat: 0.9 g saturated fat: 0.2 g cholesterol: 0 mg
sodium: 683 mg carbohydrates: 48 g dietary fiber: 8.6 g**

Finnish Vegetable Soup

This may be the best soup you've ever tasted.

2 C	water	500 mL
2 C	low-fat chicken broth	500 mL
1 C	green beans, cut into small pieces	250 mL
1 C	carrots, sliced thinly	250 mL
1 C	potatoes, diced	250 mL
1 C	peas, fresh or frozen	250 mL
1 C	cauliflower florets	250 mL
½ C	spinach, chopped	125 mL
3 T	flour	45 mL
4 C	fat-free milk	1 L
1 T	butter or margarine	15 mL
4 T	fresh parsley, chopped	60 mL

Pour the water and chicken broth into a large saucepan. Bring to a boil. Add the green beans, carrots, and potatoes. Reduce heat to a simmer and cook for 10 minutes. Add the peas, cauliflower florets, and spinach. Cook until the cauliflower is tender when pierced with a fork. In a bowl, mix the flour with one cup (250 mL) of the milk. Stir until smooth. Add the flour mixture to the soup. Add remaining milk and simmer for 10 minutes. Stir in butter and parsley.

Yield: 6 servings

Each serving contains:
**calories: 155 total fat: 2.6 g saturated fat:1.4 g cholesterol: 0.8 mg
sodium: 237 mg carbohydrates: 24.2 g dietary fiber: 3.9 g**

Cold Cuke Soup

Do cucumbers bother you? This low-fat cooked cucumber soup is a
friend of folks with stomach problems, not an enemy. It's worth trying.

2 T	butter or margarine	30 mL
½	medium onion, chopped	½
3	large cucumbers, peeled, with seeds discarded, chopped	3
3 T	flour	45 mL
2 C	low-fat chicken broth	500 mL
¾ C	fat-free sour cream	185 mL
1 T	fresh dill, chopped	15 mL
½ t	mace	2 mL
½ t	grated lemon rind	2 mL

In a large saucepan or Dutch oven, melt the butter. Add the chopped onion and cucumber. Sauté until tender. Sprinkle the flour over the mixture, and then add the chicken broth. Cover and simmer for 20 minutes. Cool. Puree in a blender or food processor. Stir in the remaining ingredients. Chill at least 4 hours before serving.

Yield: 6 servings

Each serving contains:
**calories: 99 total fat: 4.3 g saturated fat: 2.5 g cholesterol: 10 mg
sodium: 209 mg carbohydrates: 11.5 g dietary fiber: 1.6 g**

Vichyssoise

A low-fat version of the famous French potato soup.

6	medium potatoes, peeled and diced	6
3 T	butter or margarine	45 mL
6 stalks	leeks, sliced and washed thoroughly	6 stalks
8 C	low-fat chicken broth	2 L
2 C	nonfat sour cream	500 mL

In a covered saucepan, bring the potatoes to a boil. Lower heat and cook until the potatoes are fork-tender. Drain and set aside. In a frying pan, melt the butter, add the leeks, and sauté until they begin to get limp. Add 2 cups (500 mL) of chicken broth and continue cooking the leeks until they are soft. Put the potatoes and leeks into a food processor or blender. (You don't need to add all the chicken broth, but save any you don't put into the food processor.) Blend thoroughly, combine with the rest of the chicken broth, and chill for 24 hours. Before serving, add the sour cream and stir to combine.

Yield: 6 servings

Each serving contains:
**calories: 288 total fat: 6.2 g saturated fat: 3.6 g cholesterol: 15 mg
sodium: 539 mg carbohydrates: 47 g dietary fiber: 4.0 g**

Summer Green Bean Soup

An elegant soup for a hot summer day.

1 lb.	green beans, trimmed, cut into 1 inch (2.5 cm) pieces	454 g
2	egg yolks, beaten lightly	2
3 T	flour	45 mL
1 T	lemon juice (fresh is best)	15 mL
⅓ C	fat-free sour cream (optional)	80 mL

Cook the beans in 1½ quarts (1.5 L) of boiling water. Drain, reserving 5 cups (1.25 L) of the cooking water. Refrigerate the beans. In the empty saucepan combine the egg yolks and flour. Stir in the lemon juice. Using a wire whisk add the reserved cooking liquid a little at a time over low heat. When all the liquid has been added, simmer over medium heat until the soup thickens. Cool, and chill, adding beans. Serve cold. Garnish with a dollop of sour cream, if desired.

Yield: 6 servings

Each serving contains:
**calories: 59 total fat: 1.8 g saturated fat: 0.6 g cholesterol: 71 mg
sodium: 7 mg carbohydrates: 9.0 g dietary fiber: 2.6 g**

Chapter 4
SIDE DISHES

Russian Salad

Don't be put off by the long list of ingredients. This is both a potato dish and a vegetable dish! Make it in the summer to serve with barbecue.

1 T	olive oil	15 mL
2 cloves	garlic, minced	2 cloves
1 t	lemon juice (fresh is best)	5 mL
20	small, red potatoes, washed and cut in quarters	20
12	carrots, peeled and cut into coins	12
½ lb.	green beans, cut into 1 inch (2.5 cm) pieces	225 g
2	small zucchini, cut into chunks	2
1	small summer squash cut into chunks	1
¼ C	wine vinegar or raspberry vinegar	60 mL
1 T	water	15 mL
1 bunch	scallions, chopped	1 bunch
¼ t	pepper (optional)	2 mL
6	leaves of lettuce for serving (optional)	6

Stir the olive oil, minced garlic, and lemon juice together in a small bowl and set aside. Place potatoes and carrots in a steamer basket and cook over boiling water for 8-10 minutes. Add the beans, zucchini, and squash and steam for 3-5 minutes longer. Don't overcook. The vegetables should still be crispy, but tender. Put the vegetables into a large bowl. Using a fork, mix the vinegar and water together in a small bowl or cup. Sprinkle the scallions over the vegetables. Spoon 2 T (30 mL) of the vinegar and water mixture over the hot vegetables. Using two large spoons, toss the vegetables gently. Set aside for 15 minutes. Pour the remaining mixture into the oil mixture, and add the pepper, if desired. Use a fork to mix well. Drizzle over the vegetables. Toss again gently. Serve on lettuce leaves, if desired.

Yield: 10 servings

Each serving contains:
  calories: 241 total fat: 1.8 g saturated fat: 0.3 g cholesterol: 0 mg
  sodium: 46 mg carbohydrates: 52.6 g dietary fiber: 7.5 g

Macaroni Salad

Best when made early in the day so that the flavors can blend by dinnertime.

4 oz.	dry macaroni	100 g
2 T	water	30 mL
⅓ C	fat-free mayonnaise	80 mL
1	small onion or scallion, diced	1
3 T	cider vinegar	45 mL
2 t	celery seed	10 mL
1 t	dry mustard (optional)	5 mL
1 T	sugar	15 mL
6 T	green or red pepper, finely diced	90 mL
dash	white pepper (optional)	dash
¼ t	onion powder (optional)	2 mL
4	lettuce leaves (optional)	4

Cook the macaroni as directed on the box, but omit the salt. Drain, rinse with water, and drain again. Mix the macaroni in a bowl with all remaining ingredients. Chill. Serve on lettuce leaves, if desired.

Yield: 4 servings

Each serving contains:
  calories: 152 total fat: 0.8 g saturated fat: 0.1 g cholesterol: 9 mg
  sodium: 242 mg carbohydrates: 29.7 g dietary fiber: 1.5 g

Mushroom Salad

Make this first, refrigerate it, and then make the rest of your meal. That way the flavors will have a chance to blend before it is served.

1	medium head of Boston, or other leaf lettuce	1
½ lb.	fresh mushrooms	225 g
4 T	olive oil	60 mL
1½ T	vinegar (Balsamic and wine are good choices)	22 mL
dash	salt (optional)	dash

Break the lettuce into small pieces after it has been washed and dried. Put it into a salad bowl. Wipe the mushrooms with a damp cloth. Slice the mushrooms and add them to the lettuce in the salad bowl. In a small bowl or glass, mix the oil and vinegar. Add salt, if desired. Pour the dressing over the salad and toss to coat.

Yield: 4 servings

Each serving contains:
**calories: 152 total fat: 14.1 g saturated fat: 1.9 g cholesterol: 0 mg
sodium: 9 mg carbohydrates: 6.1 g dietary fiber: 2.0 g**

Green Bean Salad

Make this a few hours before the meal and refrigerate before serving to blend the flavors.

2 lb.	fresh green beans, ends removed	907 g
3 C	boiling water	750 mL
½ C	olive oil	125 mL
¼ C	raspberry vinegar	60 mL
1 T	sugar	15 mL
1	medium onion, diced (optional)	1

Place the green beans in a heat-tolerant bowl. Pour the boiling water over the beans. Cover and set aside for 10-15 minutes. Drain in a colander. Spread the beans on a shallow serving dish. Combine the rest of the ingredients in a food processor or blender. Blend until smooth. Pour the mixture over the beans. Cover tightly with aluminum or plastic wrap. Mix before serving.

Yield: 8 servings

Each serving contains:
calories: 162 total fat: 13.6 g saturated fat: 1..9 g cholesterol: 0 mg sodium: 10 mg carbohydrates: 10.1 g dietary fiber: 3.9 g

Potato Salad

Fat-free mayonnaise puts this potato salad on the low-acid-diet menu.

6 C	potatoes, peeled and chopped into bite-sized pieces	1.5 L
1	small onion, finely chopped	1
6 T	fat-free mayonnaise	90 mL

Place the potatoes in a saucepan covered with water and bring to a boil. Reduce heat and cook until the potatoes are tender. Drain. In a serving bowl, sprinkle the onion over the potatoes. Mix in mayonnaise until the potatoes and onions are evenly coated. Chill thoroughly.

Yield: 12 one-half cup (125 mL) servings

Each serving contains:
calories: 54 total fat: 0.1 g saturated fat: 0.3 g cholesterol: 3 mg sodium: 87 mg carbohydrates: 11.4 g dietary fiber: 1.1 g

Ambrosia Salad

Using fat-free sour cream really cuts down the calories of this perennial favorite.

1 (16 oz.) can	pineapple chunks in juice, drained	1 (454 g) can
1 C	seedless grapes	250 mL
2	medium bananas, peeled and cubed	2
1 (14 oz.) can	mandarin oranges, drained	1 (400 g) can
2 C	mini marshmallows	500 mL
1 C	coconut flakes	250 mL
8 oz.	fat-free sour cream	200 g

In a large bowl, combine everything except the sour cream. Fold in the sour cream. Refrigerate 1 hour before serving.

Yield: 6 servings

Each serving contains:
**calories: 259 total fat: 4.5 g saturated fat: 3.7 g cholesterol: 0 mg
sodium: 74 mg carbohydrates: 55 g dietary fiber: 3.6 g**

Lime Gelatin Salad

You can unmold this gelatin before serving for a festive look.

1 pkg.	lime gelatin	1 pkg.
1 C	hot water	250 mL
1 (8 oz.) can	crushed pineapple packed in juice	1 (227 g) can
1 C	fat-free cottage cheese	250 mL
1	small apple, chopped	1
¼ C	walnuts, chopped(optional)	60 mL
¼ C	celery, chopped	60 mL
8 oz.	low calorie frozen whipped topping	200 g

In a serving bowl, dissolve the lime gelatin in the hot water. Add the crushed pineapple (with its juice), cottage cheese, apple, walnuts, and celery. Mix well. Refrigerate until not quite completely set. Fold in the topping. Refrigerate until set.

Yield: 8 servings

Each serving contains:
**calories: 155 total fat: 3.6 g saturated fat: 3.6 g cholesterol: 3 mg
sodium: 106 mg carbohydrates: 18.3 g dietary fiber: 0.7 g**

Winter Fruit Salad

Try canned pears if you don't have any fresh. The recipe works just as well.

2	medium pears, cubed	2
2	bananas, sliced	2
1 C	grapes	250 mL
½ C	prunes, diced	125 mL
½ C	walnuts (optional)	125 mL
Dressing		
½	very ripe banana	½
½ C	fat-free cottage cheese	125 mL
2 T	honey	30 mL
½ C	fat-free yogurt	125 mL

Combine the fruit in one bowl and mix the dressing ingredients together in another bowl. Just before serving, toss the fruit in the dressing.

Yield: 6 servings

Each serving contains:
**calories: 176 total fat: 0.7 g saturated fat: 0.2 g cholesterol: 2 mg
sodium: 66 mg carbohydrates: 43 g dietary fiber: 4.0 g**

Waldorf Salad

Everyone's favorite!

2	medium apples, peeled, cored and coarsely chopped	2
1 T	lemon juice	15 mL
⅓ C	chopped dates	80 mL
⅓ C	raisins	80 mL
½ C	fat-free mayonnaise	125 mL

Combine the apples and lemon juice by tossing gently in a medium bowl. Add the dates and raisins, and then stir in the mayonnaise to coat the fruit evenly. Chill before serving.

Yield: 6 servings

Each serving contains:
**calories: 98 total fat: 0.3 g saturated fat: 0 g cholesterol: 9 mg
sodium: 102 mg carbohydrates: 23.0 g dietary fiber: 2.3 g**

Carrot-Raisin Salad

The color of this dish brightens up a meal.

½ C	fat-free mayonnaise	125 mL
1 T	sugar	15 mL
2 C	shredded carrots	500 mL
½ C	raisins	125 mL

In a medium bowl combine the mayonnaise and sugar until well mixed. Add the carrots and raisins. Stir and toss gently until the carrots and raisins are coated evenly.

Yield: 6 servings

Each serving contains:
**calories: 94 total fat: 0.2 g saturated fat: 0 g cholesterol: 9 mg
sodium: 127 mg carbohydrates: 21 g dietary fiber: 2.6 g**

Baked Stuffed Onions

These can be made a day ahead. Bake for 30 minutes, cover, and refrigerate. Add the cheese and finish the baking the next day.

6	medium white onions	6
2 T	butter or margarine	30 mL
1 T	water	15 mL
1 (4 oz.) can	mushrooms, drained and chopped	1 (114 g) can
1 T	pecans, finely chopped (optional)	15 mL
dash	salt	dash
1 C	low-fat beef broth	250 mL
½ C	low-fat Cheddar cheese, grated	125 mL

Peel the onions and, with a sharp knife, cut a center core, leaving about ½ inch (1.3 cm) on the sides and bottom. Save the part of the onion that was removed. Put the cored onions in a medium saucepan, fill with water, and simmer until onions are barely tender (about 10-15 minutes). Drain and set aside. Chop the reserved uncooked onion. Melt the butter in a frying pan over low heat. Stir in the water, uncooked onion, mushrooms, and pecans. Sauté 10 minutes or so. Add salt, if desired. Set the onion shells in a baking pan. (A lasagna pan lined with foil makes for easy clean-up.) Spoon the mushroom mixture into the shells. Pour the beef broth around the onions at their base. Bake in a preheated 350°F (180°C) oven for 30 minutes. Sprinkle the grated Cheddar cheese over the top of each onion. Bake 30 minutes more.

Yield: 3 servings (makes six onions)

Each two-onion serving contains:
**calories: 192 total fat: 9.3 g saturated fat: 5.7 g cholesterol: 28 mg
sodium: 1814* mg carbohydrates: 14.6 g dietary fiber: 4.3 g**

*Using beef cubes and low-salt cheese can reduce the sodium level significantly.

Summer Squash Treat

Make this in the late summer when summer squash is at its best.

1 T	butter or margarine	15 mL
¼ C	water	60 mL
⅓ C	onion, finely chopped	80 mL
2 lb.	summer squash, cut in thick slices	900 g
1 C	fat-free sour cream	250 mL
4 t	flour	20 mL

Melt the butter in a saucepan, add the water, onions, and squash. Cook until the squash is tender. In a small bowl, combine the sour cream and flour. Add this mixture to the squash and bring to a boil. Remove from heat.

Yield: 6 servings

Each serving contains:

calories: 82 total fat: 2.2 g saturated fat: 1.3 g cholesterol: 5 mg sodium: 89 mg carbohydrates: 12 g dietary fiber: 3.0 g

Zucchini Pancakes

Wonderful served with soup for a simple meal.

2	eggs or equivalent egg substitute	2
3–4 T	flour	45–60 mL
2 T	grated Parmesan cheese	30 mL
1 T	parsley, chopped	15 mL
1 t	onion powder (optional)	5 mL
3	medium zucchini, shredded	3
8 oz.	fat-free sour cream	200 g

Combine eggs, 3 T (45 mL) flour, Parmesan, parsley, and onion powder, if desired. Add zucchini. Stir. Add the remaining flour if the batter is thin. Heat a nonstick frying pan or griddle until a drop of water "dances" on it. Drop the batter by tablespoons onto the heated surface. Cook until the tops are bubbly and the bottom is browned. Flip and cook until both sides are browned. Serve hot with a dollop of sour cream on each pancake, if desired.

Yield: 4 servings

Each serving contains:
calories: 125 total fat: 3.5 g saturated fat: 1.3 g cholesterol: 108 mg sodium: 134 mg carbohydrates: 14.1 g dietary fiber: 1.3 g

Potato Pancakes

A delicious addition to any meal, but especially good with plain meats such as pork chops. Serve hot and top with applesauce.

3	medium potatoes, peeled and diced	3
1	small onion	1
1 T	flour	15 mL
1	egg or egg substitute	1
2 T	skim milk	30 mL
1 T	butter or margarine	15 mL

Preheat a griddle or frying pan over medium heat. Put the potatoes and onion into a blender or food processor, sprinkle with flour, add the egg and milk, and blend just enough to mix (too much blending will liquefy the potatoes). Melt a small amount of the butter in a frying pan. Spoon the batter onto the hot frying pan, about ¼ cup (60 mL) for each pancake. When the pancakes are brown around the edges, turn them over and cook on the other side. Add additional butter to the frying pan as needed to fry the remaining pancakes.

Yield: 8 pancakes

Each pancake contains:
calories: 63 total fat: 2.1 g saturated fat: 1.1 g cholesterol: 30 mg sodium: 95 mg carbohydrates: 9.3 g dietary fiber: 0.9 g

Parsley Potatoes

A nice way to serve potatoes when you're serving meat without gravy or sauce.

4	medium potatoes, halved or quartered	4
2 T	butter or margarine	30 mL
1	clove garlic, crushed	1
dash	dry mustard	dash
2 T	parsley, chopped fresh	30 mL
½ t	lemon juice	3 mL
grind	fresh pepper (optional)	grind

Place the potatoes in a saucepan with cold water to cover and cook over high heat until they start to boil. Lower heat and cook gently until fork-tender, 15 to 20 minutes. Melt the butter or margarine in a saucepan and remove from heat. Stir in the garlic, mustard, parsley, lemon juice, and pepper. Let stand until the potatoes are done (this will increase the flavor). Before serving, gently reheat the butter mixture and pour over the potatoes.

Yield: 4 servings

Each serving contains:
  **calories: 145 total fat: 5.9 g saturated fat: 3.6 g cholesterol: 15 mg
  sodium: 73 mg carbohydrates: 21.4 g dietary fiber: 2.0 g**

Eggplant Normande

This is a variation of a French regional dish. It's a very nice way to introduce eggplant to a skeptical eater.

2 (about 2 lb.)	medium eggplants, peeled and cubed	2 (about 1 k)
1 T	butter or margarine	15 mL
2	medium onions, diced	2

| 1 C | applesauce | 250 mL |
| ½ t | marjoram | 3 mL |

Put the eggplant in a saucepan, cover with water, and boil until tender. Pour into a colander to drain the water. Press on the eggplant with the back of a spoon to remove as much water as possible. In a frying pan, melt the butter and sauté the onions until soft and golden. In a bowl, mash the eggplant, stir in the onions, applesauce, and marjoram.

Yield: 6 servings

Each serving contains:
**calories: 98 total fat: 2.3 g saturated fat: 1.3 g cholesterol: 5 mg
sodium: 208 mg carbohydrates: 19.7 g dietary fiber: 5.0 g**

Grilled Eggplant

Grill this outdoors. Use a vegetable screen for grilling the eggplant.

¼ C	seasoned bread crumbs	60 mL
1	medium eggplant, cut into ¾ inch (2 cm) slices	1
2 T	olive oil	30 mL

Brush both sides of each slice of eggplant with the olive oil and then press each side onto bread crumbs to coat. Grill 10 to 15 minutes, turning once. The eggplant will be tender.

Yield: 4 servings

Each serving contains:
**calories: 117 total fat: 7.2 g saturated fat: 1.0 g cholesterol: 0 mg
sodium: 202 mg carbohydrates: 12.2 g dietary fiber: 2.9 g**

Thanksgiving Gelatin

Buy extra cranberries around Thanksgiving and freeze them.

1	envelope unflavored gelatin	1
½ C	water	125 mL
2 C	cranberries	500 mL
1 C	water	250 mL
½ C	corn syrup	125 mL
¼ C	sugar	60 mL
½ C	apple, peeled, cored and chopped	125 mL

Sprinkle the gelatin over the ½ C (125 mL) water. Set aside. In a saucepan, combine the cranberries, the 1 C (250 mL) water, corn syrup, and sugar. Heat over medium heat, stirring constantly, until the cranberries begin to pop. Remove from heat. Stir the gelatin mixture into the hot cranberry mixture. Fold in the chopped apple. Turn the mixture into a serving bowl. Chill until firm.

Yield: 6 servings

Each serving contains:
**calories: 178 total fat: 0.1 g saturated fat: 0 g cholesterol: 0 mg
sodium: 62 mg carbohydrates: 34.7 g dietary fiber: 12.3 g**

Sweet & Sour Red Cabbage

This is great as a leftover, too.

4 T	sugar	60 mL
4 T	olive oil	60 mL
1	medium onion, sliced	1
1	medium red cabbage, cored and shredded	1
2	apples, peeled, sliced and cored	2
4 T	vinegar	60 mL
1 C	water (optional dry red wine)	250 mL

In a large saucepan that has a tightly fitting cover, combine the sugar and oil. Cook together over moderate heat until the mixture is caramel-colored. Reduce heat and add the onion. Stir frequently, cooking until the onion is soft and golden. Stir in the rest of the ingredients. Bring to a boil and cover. Reduce heat to low and simmer for 40 minutes. Taste before serving, and add a little more sugar, if needed.) Serve warm.

Yield: 10 servings

Each serving contains:
calories: 111 total fat: 5.8 g saturated fat: 0.8 g cholesterol: 0 mg sodium: 65 mg carbohydrates: 15.7 g dietary fiber: 1.4 g

Asparagus with Soy Dressing

The soy dressing adds an exotic taste to the asparagus.

1 lb.	fresh asparagus (thin is best)	450 g
2 t	olive oil	10 mL
2 t	soy sauce	10 mL
1½ t	sugar	8 mL

Cut off the white ends of the asparagus and slice the stalks diagonally into 2 inch (5 cm) pieces. Wash and set aside. In a large, heavy-bottomed skillet, heat the oil over medium heat. Add the asparagus and, stirring constantly, fry for a minute or two until the asparagus becomes tender. Sprinkle the soy sauce over the asparagus and stir-fry for another minute. Sprinkle the sugar over the vegetable mixture and stir-fry 30 seconds more. Turn into a serving bowl.

Yield: 4 servings

Each serving contains:
calories: 53 total fat: 2.5 g saturated fat: 0.4 g cholesterol: 0 mg sodium: 140 mg carbohydrates: 6.9 g dietary fiber: 2.4 g

Parsnips? Parsnips!

Parsnips are often overlooked today, but they are actually a very sweet and good vegetable. This is a great recipe for getting acquainted with parsnips.

2 lb.	parsnips, scraped and trimmed	900 g
2 T	brown sugar	30 mL
½ t	dry mustard	3 mL
2 T	butter or margarine	30 mL

Cut the parsnips lengthwise into strips. In a medium saucepan, heat 1 inch (2.5 cm) of water to boiling. Put in the parsnips and cover. Cook until tender, about 25 minutes. Drain in a colander. Arrange in a lasagna pan. In a small bowl or cup, mix together the brown sugar and mustard. Sprinkle this mixture over the parsnips and dot with butter. Bake in a preheated 400°F (200°C) oven for about 20 minutes. The parsnips will be glazed and light brown.

Yield: 8 servings

Each serving contains:
    **calories: 119 total fat: 3.2 g saturated fat: 1.8 g cholesterol: 8 mg
    sodium: 41 mg carbohydrates: 22.6 g dietary fiber: 5.6 g**

Baked Acorn Squash

Acorn squash, the easiest of all squashes to prepare, is a good choice when your oven is on for other dishes, or even by itself.

2	large acorn squashes (more if they're small)	2
4 T	maple syrup	60 mL
4 t	butter or margarine	20 mL

Cut the squash in half, remove the seeds and stringy part to make a well in the center, and put the halves on a cookie sheet, cut side up.

Add 1 T maple syrup and 1 t butter in each well. (Some cooks like to substitute another syrup or brown sugar.) Bake in 400°F (200°C) oven until soft when pierced with a fork.

Yield: 4 servings.

Each serving contains:
calories: 238 total fat: 11.6 g saturated fat: 7.1 g cholesterol: 31 mg sodium: 124 mg carbohydrates: 35.7 g dietary fiber: 0 g

Sweet Potatoes & Apples

A sweet side dish in the Southern style.

2 (17 oz.) cans	vacuum-packed sweet potatoes	2 (460 g) cans
2	medium cooking apples, peeled, cored and sliced	2
¼ C	molasses	60 mL
2 T	sugar	30 mL
2 T	butter or margarine, melted	30 mL
⅓ C	orange juice	80 mL
½ t	cinnamon (optional)	3 mL

Cut each piece of sweet potato in half. Arrange the sweet potatoes and apples in an ungreased baking pan (the kind used for brownies works well). In a small bowl, mix together the rest of the ingredients and pour the mixture over the apples and potatoes. Do not cover. Bake in a preheated 350°F (180°C) oven for 35-45 minutes. The apples will be tender but not mushy.

Yield: 8 servings

Each serving contains:
calories: 216 total fat: 3.4 g saturated fat: 1.9 g cholesterol: 8 mg sodium: 49 mg carbohydrates: 45.8 g dietary fiber: 4.6 g

Sweet Potato Puffs

Ramekins are small ceramic soufflé dishes. Get some for this recipe and use them to serve individual portions of pudding, fruit salad, gelatin, and the like.

2 C	canned sweet potatoes, drained	500 mL
1	ripe banana, mashed	1
1½ T	olive oil	22 mL
1	egg yolk	1
1½ t	salt (optional)	8 mL
¼ C	milk, heated until hot	60 mL
1	egg white, beaten stiff	1

Process the sweet potatoes in a blender or food processor. Transfer to a mixing bowl. Beat in the banana, olive oil, egg yolk, salt (if desired), and then the milk. Using a rubber scraper, fold in the egg white. Divide into 12 ramekins coated with nonstick cooking spray. Bake in a preheated 500°F (250°C) oven for 12 minutes.

Yield: 12 puffs

Each puff contains:
**calories: 55.9 total fat: 2.4 g saturated fat: 0.5 g cholesterol: 18 mg
sodium: 11 mg carbohydrates: 7.8 g dietary fiber: 0.9 g**

Baked Glazed Yams

Easy enough for an everyday meal and fancy enough for company.

1 (17 oz.) can	yams or sweet potatoes	1 (460 g) can
1	ripe banana	1
¼ C	sugar	60 mL
1 t	cinnamon (optional)	5 mL
2 T	lemon juice	30 mL
½ C	molasses	125 mL

Mash together the yams, banana, sugar, cinnamon, and lemon juice. Spoon into a small casserole and drizzle molasses over the top. Bake in a 350°F (180°C) oven for 15-20 minutes. The mixture will be bubbly.

Yield: 4 servings

Each serving contains:
calories: 295 total fat: 0.4 g saturated fat: 0.1 g cholesterol: 0 mg sodium: 80 mg carbohydrates: 73.5 g dietary fiber: 4.3 g

French Carrots Supreme

When you slice carrots on the diagonal they look fancy and festive. But the recipe is really quite simple.

1 T	butter or margarine	15 mL
¾ C	low-fat chicken broth	185 mL
2 t	sugar	10 mL
5 C	diagonally sliced carrots	1.25 L
2 t	lemon juice	10 mL
¼ C	chopped parsley	60 mL

Add the butter to the chicken broth in the saucepan. Bring to a boil. Add the sugar and carrots. Lower heat to a simmer, cover, and cook until carrots are tender when a fork is inserted, about 10 minutes or so. Stir in lemon juice and parsley.

Yield: 6 servings

Each serving contains:
calories: 107 total fat: 2.3 g saturated fat: 1.2 g cholesterol: 5 mg sodium: 128 mg carbohydrates: 20.8 g dietary fiber: 5.5 g

Macaroni, Corn and Cheese Casserole

Great as a leftover, too.

½ C	egg noodles	125 mL
1	egg, or equivalent egg substitute, lightly beaten	1
½ C	low-fat Cheddar cheese, grated	125 mL
1 C	cream-style corn	250 mL
½ C	bread crumbs	125 mL
1 T	butter or margarine	15 mL

Cook the egg noodles in boiling water, and drain. Mix together with the egg, cheese, and corn. Transfer to a 1 quart (1 liter) baking dish. Sprinkle the bread crumbs over the top. Dot with butter. Bake in a preheated 350°F (180°C) oven for 30 minutes.

Yield: 4 servings

Each serving contains:
**calories: 306 total fat: 8.1 g saturated fat: 3.4 g cholesterol: 68 mg
sodium: 241 mg carbohydrates: 44.5 g dietary fiber: 0.8 g**

Corn Pudding

Tastes like the old-fashioned kind Grandma made.

2 C	frozen corn kernels	500 mL
1½ C	skim milk	375 mL
2 T	butter or margarine, melted	30 mL
1 T	sugar	15 mL
3	eggs or equivalent egg substitute, lightly beaten	3

Coat a 1½ quart (1.5 L) casserole with nonstick cooking spray. Combine the ingredients and turn into the casserole. Place the casserole in a pan of hot water. Bake in a preheated 350°F (180°C) oven for 45 minutes or until the pudding is set.

Yield: 4 servings

Each serving contains:
**calories: 222 total fat: 10.2 g saturated fat: 4.9 g cholesterol: 176 mg
sodium: 155 mg carbohydrates: 25.1 g dietary fiber: 2.0 g**

Creamy Corn

Rich and creamy, fat-free cream cheese and milk cut the calories.

¼ C	fat-free milk	60 mL
3 oz.	fat-free cream cheese	85 g
1 T	butter or margarine	15 mL
½ t	salt (optional)	3 mL
3 C	canned corn, drained	750 mL

In a saucepan, combine the milk, cream cheese, butter and salt, if desired. Warm over low heat, stirring constantly, until the cheese is melted and mixture is blended. Add corn, stir and heat.

Yield: 6 servings

Each serving contains:
**calories: 111 total fat: 2.5 g saturated fat: 1.3 g cholesterol: 8 mg
sodium: 416 mg carbohydrates: 21 g dietary fiber: 1.0 g**

Creamy Carrots

Use frozen carrots if you like. Cook according to package directions, drain and add the other ingredients.

8	medium carrots, peeled, and quartered lengthwise	8
1 t	sugar	5 mL
3 T	fat-free mayonnaise	45 mL
2 T	fat-free sour cream	30 mL

Put carrots into boiling water with sugar. Cover and cook until tender, 15-20 minutes. Drain. In a serving dish, mix together the mayonnaise and sour cream. Add the carrots and toss to mix lightly.

Yield: 6 servings

Each serving contains:
   **calories: 55 total fat: 0.2 g saturated fat: 0 g cholesterol: 3 mg
   sodium: 76 mg carbohydrates: 11.8 g dietary fiber: 2.9 g**

Creamy Peas

The chicken broth adds a rich taste to ordinary peas.

¼ C	low-fat chicken broth	60 mL
10 oz.	frozen peas	284 g
4 T	fat-free sour cream	60 mL

Heat the chicken broth in a small saucepan. Stir in the frozen peas and cook until tender. Drain. Spoon the sour cream over the peas. Toss lightly to combine.

Yield: 4 servings

Each serving contains:
   **calories: 61 total fat: 0.3 g saturated fat: 0.1 g cholesterol: 0 mg
   sodium: 25 mg carbohydrates: 10.7 g dietary fiber: 3.6 g**

Cucumbers in Sour Cream

A traditional favorite.

| 2 | medium-sized cucumbers | 2 |
| ½ C | nonfat sour cream | 125 mL |

Peel the cucumbers and cut them into very thin slices. Cover with the sour cream and refrigerate for an hour or two before serving.

Yield: 4 servings

Each serving contains:
**calories: 40 total fat: 0.2 g saturated fat: 0.1 g cholesterol: 0 mg
sodium: 28 mg carbohydrates: 7.2 g dietary fiber: 1.2 g**

Green Beans with Sour Cream

Sour cream transforms frozen green beans into a gourmet dish.

1 (10 oz.) pkg.	frozen green beans	1 (284 g) pkg.
4 T	nonfat sour cream	60 mL
1 T	grated Parmesan cheese	15 mL

Cook beans in boiling water according to package directions. Drain. Stir in sour cream. Transfer to a serving dish and sprinkle with cheese.

Yield: 4 servings

Each serving contains:
**calories: 38 total fat: 0.5 g saturated fat: 0.3 g cholesterol: 1 mg
sodium: 40 mg carbohydrates: 6.7 g dietary fiber: 2.4 g**

Chapter 5
MAIN DISHES

Baked Cod or Haddock

Even people who don't usually like fish ask for seconds of this traditional New England "Baked Scrod" recipe.

1½ lb.	fresh cod or haddock	700 g
3 T	lemon juice	45 mL
½ C	bread crumbs	125 mL
2 T	butter or margarine	30 mL

Place fish, one piece deep, in a lasagna pan (13 x 9 x 2 in, or 33 x 23 x 5 cm). Sprinkle the lemon juice over the fish. Then sprinkle the bread crumbs evenly over the top. Dot with butter. Bake in a preheated 350°F (180°C) oven for 30 minutes or so, until fish flakes evenly.

Yield: 4 servings

Each serving contains:
calories: 353 total fat: 13.6 g saturated fat: 4.6 g cholesterol: 15 mg sodium: 84 mg carbohydrates: 49.6 g dietary fiber: 4.0 g

Pan-Fried Fish Fillets

Use a nonstick frying pan to cut down on the amount of fat needed.

1 lb.	fish fillets (ocean perch, haddock, or flounder)	450 g
2 t	butter or margarine	10 mL
2 t	canola oil	10 mL
⅓ C	bread crumbs	80 mL
¼ C	skim milk	60 mL

Wash fillets and pat dry. In a frying pan, melt some of the butter, and some of the oil. Spread out the bread crumbs on a plate. Put the milk into a wide bowl. Dip the fish into the milk to moisten. Coat the fish with bread crumbs by placing the fish on the bread crumbs, one side at a time. Fry in the butter/oil mixture for 4 or 5 minutes on each side. Add more butter and oil to the frying pan as needed. Serve with Quick Cucumber Sauce.

Yield: 4 servings

Each serving contains:
**calories: 205 total fat: 9.6 g saturated fat: 4.0 g cholesterol: 64 mg
sodium: 190 mg carbohydrates: 7.4 g dietary fiber: 0.5 g**

Broiled Marinated Fish or Shrimp

As good as any in a restaurant. Great with pasta or rice and a salad.

2 T	olive oil	30 mL
1 T	parsley, finely chopped	15 mL
¼ C	lemon juice	60 mL
2	cloves garlic, chopped	2
1 C	white wine	250 mL
⅛ t	black or white pepper	1 mL
1 lb.	boneless fish fillets or shrimp, cleaned	450 g

Mix the oil, parsley, lemon juice, garlic, wine, and pepper in a non-metallic bowl. Put the fish fillets into the marinade and refrigerate for at least two hours. Preheat the broiler and brush the hot rack with the marinade. Broil close to the heat for approximately 5 minutes until the fish flakes when touched with a fork; broil shrimp about 3 minutes.

Yield: 4 servings

Each serving contains:
**calories: 202 total fat: 7.6 g saturated fat: 1.1 g cholesterol: 49 mg
sodium: 69 mg carbohydrates: 2.8 g dietary fiber: 0.2 g**

Parsley Scallops

This is a super make-ahead summer recipe. Serve with macaroni or potato salad and a tossed salad with fat-free dressing.

1 slice	onion	1 slice
1 slice	lemon	1 slice
2 C	water	500 mL
1 lb.	scallops	450 g
2 T	fat-free bottled Italian salad dressing	30 mL
½ C	parsley, chopped	125 mL

Combine the onion and lemon slices in the water in a medium saucepan. Heat until the water begins to boil. Add the scallops. Remove from the heat. Cover and let stand for 5 minutes. Drain. In a small mixing bowl, combine the salad dressing and parsley. Add the scallops and toss. Cover and chill until serving.

Yield: 2 servings

Each serving contains:
  **calories: 286 total fat: 2.7 g saturated fat: 0.3 g cholesterol: 75 mg
    sodium: 709 mg carbohydrates: 24.9 g dietary fiber: 2.5 g**

Scallops with Snow Peas

Frozen snow peas are fine if you can't get any fresh ones.

½ lb.	snow peas	225 g
¼ C	water	60 mL
½ C	sweet pepper, diced	125 mL
1 T	butter or margarine	15 mL
1 T	olive oil	15 mL
¾ lb.	scallops	340 g
½ t	salt (optional)	3 mL

Trim the peas by cutting off the stem end. Place them in a large skillet that has a tightly fitting cover, add the water, and cook, covered, for 2 minutes or so. Take the cover off and cook for a minute or so more. Add the sweet pepper, butter, and oil. Stir in the scallops and sauté over very high heat for 2 to 4 minutes. Serve at once.

Yield: 4 servings

Each serving contains:
  **calories: 157 total fat: 7.1 g saturated fat: 2.4 g cholesterol: 36 mg
  sodium: 300 mg carbohydrates: 6.8 g dietary fiber: 1.8 g**

Creamed Shrimp with Peas

Serve over rice or toast.

2 T	butter or margarine	30 mL
¼ C	onion, diced very fine	60 mL
4 T	flour	60 mL
1 C	nonfat milk	250 mL
1 C	evaporated skim milk	250 mL
1 C	shrimp (fresh or canned, drained if canned)	250 mL
1 C	peas (frozen are fine)	250 mL
1 t	lemon juice	5 mL
1 t	sherry	5 mL

Melt the butter in a saucepan, add the onion, and cook over low heat until the onion is soft and translucent. Sprinkle the flour over the butter and onions and cook a few minutes. Gradually stir in the two kinds of milk and heat gently, stirring constantly until the sauce is thickened. Add the shrimp and peas, lemon juice and sherry. Heat thoroughly.

Yield: 2 servings

Each serving contains:
**calories: 417 total fat: 13.1 g saturated fat: 7.6 g cholesterol: 113 mg
  sodium: 476 mg carbohydrates: 44.2 g dietary fiber: 4.0 g**

Finnish Baked Salmon Dinner

Although this is usually made with salmon, try other firm fish you like.

2 lb.	salmon	900 g
2 T	butter or margarine	30 mL
1 C	onions, diced	250 mL
1½ lb.	potatoes, peeled and thickly sliced	700 g
1 t	salt (optional)	5 mL
3 T	bread crumbs	45 mL
2	eggs, or equivalent egg substitute	2
2 C	nonfat milk	500 mL

Wash the salmon, pat dry, and cut into small (bite size) pieces. In a frying pan, melt the butter. Add the onions and sauté a few minutes until the onions are soft. Spray a two quart (2 L) baking dish with nonstick cooking spray. Put a layer of potatoes on the bottom of the dish, then a layer of salmon and onions. Sprinkle with salt, if desired. Make the last layer a potato layer. Sprinkle the bread crumbs over the top. In a small bowl, beat the eggs and milk together and then pour this mixture into the baking dish. Bake in a preheated 350°F (180°C) oven for 1 hour.

Yield: 6 servings

Each serving contains:
**calories: 308 total fat: 11.9 g saturated fat: 4.1 g cholesterol: 197 mg
sodium: 337 mg carbohydrates: 11.2 g dietary fiber: 0.8 g**

Crab Asparagus au Gratin

This only takes 15 minutes to bake in a preheated oven and is fairly easy to prepare.

20 oz.	frozen asparagus, cooked and diced	570 g
2	slices high-fiber bread, crumbed in a blender	2
⅔ C	nonfat dry milk powder	170 mL
⅓ C	Parmesan cheese, grated	80 mL
1¾ C	boiling water	440 mL
2 T	butter or margarine, softened	30 mL
1	egg or equivalent egg substitute, lightly beaten	1
13 oz.	crabmeat	370 g

Arrange cooked and drained asparagus in a shallow baking dish. In a blender or food processor combine the bread crumbs, milk powder, and about half the Parmesan cheese and half the boiling water. During the processing add the remaining water, the butter, and the egg. Wash the crabmeat, break up any large pieces, and remove any crab shells or cartilage. Pour the sauce from the blender or food processor or bowl over the crabmeat. Stir. Pour this mixture over the asparagus. Sprinkle the remaining Parmesan on top. Bake in a preheated 400°F (200°C) oven for 15 minutes.

Yield: 6 servings

Each serving contains:
**calories: 211 total fat: 7.2 g saturated fat: 3.7 g cholesterol: 100 mg
sodium: 385 mg carbohydrates: 15.2 g dietary fiber: 2.3 g**

Baked Seafood Casserole

This is a low-fat version of President Kennedy's favorite recipe.

1 lb.	crabmeat	450 g
1 lb.	shrimp, cooked and peeled	450 g
1 C	fat-free mayonnaise	250 mL
¼ C	onion, minced	60 mL
1½ C	celery, finely chopped (optional)	375 mL
1 T	Worcestershire sauce	15 mL
2 C	crushed baked potato chips	500 mL

Mix all the ingredients together except the potato chips. Transfer to a baking pan and cover the top with the crushed potato chips. Bake in a preheated 400°F (200°C) oven for 20-25 minutes.

Yield: 12 servings

Each serving contains:
calories: 108 total fat: 1.1 g saturated fat: 0.2 g cholesterol: 100 mg sodium: 310 mg carbohydrates: 5.2 g dietary fiber: 0.2 g

Sunday Night "Clamlet"

Wonderful served with soup and bread, and not just for the weekend.

2 T	butter or margarine	30 mL
2 T	water	30 mL
1	medium onion, diced	1
4	cooked potatoes, peeled and chopped	4
4	eggs, or egg substitute, lightly beaten	4
4 T	fat-free sour cream	60 mL
4 T	Parmesan cheese, grated	60 mL
13 oz.	clams, drained and chopped	368 g

Melt the butter in a frying pan, add the water and onions, and sauté until the onions are soft. Add the potatoes and fry to brown the potatoes. In a bowl, beat together the eggs, sour cream, and cheese. Sprinkle the clams on top of the potatoes in the frying pan. Pour the egg mixture over everything and cook over low heat another 10 minutes or so, until the eggs are set.

Yield: 4 servings

Each serving contains:
**calories: 264 total fat: 12.5 g saturated fat: 6.1 g cholesterol: 237 mg
sodium: 378 mg carbohydrates: 24 g dietary fiber: 2.3 g**

Macaroni and Tuna Salad

A summer favorite.

1 lb.	elbow macaroni, cooked	450 g
½ C	finely diced onion	125 mL
1 C	frozen peas	250 mL
1 (12 oz.) can	white tuna, packed in water	1 (340 g) can
1¾ C	fat-free mayonnaise	435 mL

Combine all ingredients in a mixing bowl. Cover tightly and chill.

Yield: 16 servings

Each serving contains:
**calories: 226 total fat: 10.5 g saturated fat: 1.7 g cholesterol: 6 mg
sodium: 336 mg carbohydrates: 22.8 g dietary fiber: 1.2 g**

Vegetable and Macaroni Bake

Try your favorite vegetables instead of, or in addition to, celery and green peppers.

1 C	sweet onion or leeks, sliced thin	250 mL
2	celery stalks, chopped fine	2
1	green pepper, chopped fine (optional)	1
1 C	whole wheat macaroni, cooked	250 mL
⅔ C	nonfat yogurt	170 mL
1 C	nonfat ricotta cheese	250 mL
2 t	soy sauce	10 mL
½ C	Cheddar cheese, low-fat, shredded	125 mL

In a medium bowl, mix together the onion, celery, green pepper, and macaroni. In another bowl, combine the yogurt, ricotta, and soy sauce. Combine the contents of the two bowls. Mix well. Put into an ovenproof dish coated with nonstick cooking spray. Sprinkle the Cheddar cheese over the top. Bake in a preheated 350° (180°C) oven for 30 minutes.

Yield: 4 servings

Each serving contains:
> **calories: 217 total fat: 1.5 g saturated fat: 0.8 g cholesterol: 5 mg**
> **sodium: 451 mg carbohydrates: 37.0 g dietary fiber: 1.2 g**

Pasta Primavera

For extra fiber, use whole wheat pasta.

2 T	olive oil	30 mL
2 T	butter or margarine	30 mL
2	cloves garlic, finely minced	2
2 C	broccoli, cut into fairly small pieces	500 mL
1 C	sweet red or green peppers, cut into thin strips	250 mL
1 C	carrots, cut in strips, 1–1½ in. (2.5–4 cm) long	250 mL
8 oz.	linguine or another pasta	200 g
grind	black pepper (optional)	grind
sprinkle	garlic powder (optional)	sprinkle

Heat the oil and butter or margarine in a frying pan. Add the garlic and vegetables and cook for approximately 10 minutes. The vegetables should still have some crispness. Cook the linguine as directed on the box, but leave out the salt. Drain the linguine and, using two large spoons, toss in a large bowl with the vegetables. Grind the pepper on top and toss again. Garlic lovers will want garlic powder sprinkled on top.

Yield: 4 servings

Each serving contains:
**calories: 247 total fat: 7.7 g saturated fat: 4.0 g cholesterol: 89 mg
sodium: 244 mg carbohydrates: 10.9 g dietary fiber: 0.7 g**

Fresh Parsley Pesto and Fettuccine

This is best with fresh basil and fresh parsley. It's easy and fast to prepare.

½ t	basil, dried or double amount of fresh basil	3 mL
½ C	fresh parsley clusters	125 mL
2	large cloves garlic (optional)	2
½ C	pine nuts	125 mL
4 t	lemon juice	20 mL
4 oz.	low-fat Swiss cheese	100 g
2 t	olive oil	10 mL
8 oz.	fettuccine or egg noodles	200 g

Combine the basil, parsley, garlic, nuts, lemon juice, and cheese in the blender or food processor. Turn on the blender and slowly add the olive oil. Blend until smooth. Stop the blender and scrape down the sides. Cook the fettuccine without salt. Drain and turn into a warm bowl. Pour the sauce over the fettuccine. Serve warm.

Yield: 4 servings

Each serving contains:
calories: 412 total fat: 16.6 g saturated fat: 3.3 g cholesterol: 64 mg sodium: 120 mg carbohydrates: 48.6 g dietary fiber: 3.3 g

Potato Cheese Puff

A beautiful and tasty casserole you can throw together very quickly.

3 C	mashed potatoes	750 mL
2	eggs, or equivalent egg substitute, lightly beaten	2
1½ C	nonfat milk	375 mL
⅓ C	Parmesan cheese, grated	80 mL
4 oz.	skim mozzarella cheese, shredded	100 g
1 C	lean ham, chopped	250 mL
2 T	fresh parsley, chopped	30 mL
1 T	butter or margarine, melted	15 mL

In a medium bowl, beat the mashed potatoes and eggs. Blend in the milk gradually. Then blend in the rest of the ingredients. Spoon into an 8 inch (20 cm) square baking dish coated with a nonstick cooking spray. Sprinkle with additional Parmesan, if desired. Bake in preheated 350°F (180°C) oven for about 1 hour. The center will be firm.

Yield: 9 squares

Each square contains:
**calories: 133 total fat: 6.3 g saturated fat: 3.4 g cholesterol: 68 mg
sodium: 397 mg carbohydrates: 7.7 g dietary fiber: 0.5 g**

Potatoes Stuffed with Broccoli and Ham

Lower fat and calorie version of the fast food favorite.

4	medium potatoes, baked	4
4 T	skim milk	60 mL
1½ C	frozen cut-up broccoli	375 mL
½ C	low-fat ham	125 mL
½ C	fat-free Cheddar cheese, shredded	125 mL

Slice a two-inch (5 cm) cut into each potato on the long side. Scoop out the soft inside into a bowl leaving about ¼ inch (6 mm) against the skin. Add the milk, broccoli and diced ham to the bowl. Mix well. Add half the cheese. Stir thoroughly. Put the mixture back into the potato skins. Pile any extra outside the top of the potatoes. Bake in a preheated 375°F (190°C) oven for 25–30 minutes. As you remove the potatoes from the oven, sprinkle on the reserved cheese. Return to the oven for a minute or two to melt the cheese.

Yield: 4 stuffed potatoes

Each stuffed potato contains:
calories: 156 total fat: 2.1 g saturated fat: 0.7 g cholesterol: 13 mg sodium: 335 mg carbohydrates: 23.2 g dietary fiber: 2.8 g

Ham-Stuffed Zucchini

This is a way to use those zucchini that seem to grow overnight. Store-bought work fine, too!

8	small zucchini	8
4 C	low-fat ham, chopped fine	1 L
2	eggs or egg substitute, lightly beaten	2
1 t	basil	5 mL
½ C	green pepper, chopped (optional)	125 mL
¼ C	low-fat Swiss cheese, shredded	60 mL
1 T	canola oil	15 mL

With a sharp knife, cut off the ends of the zucchini and hollow out the inside, removing the pulp. In a mixing bowl, combine the ham, eggs, basil, green pepper (if desired) and cheese. Pack ½ cup (125 mL) of this mixture into each zucchini, using fingers or a teaspoon. Place the zucchini in a baking dish coated with a nonstick cooking spray. Brush the stuffed zucchini with the oil. Bake in a preheated 325°F (160°C) oven for 45 minutes. The zucchini will be fork-tender.

Yield: 8 servings

Each serving contains:
**calories: 190 total fat: 6.6 g saturated fat: 1.8 g cholesterol: 109 mg
sodium: 29 mg carbohydrates: 8.5 g dietary fiber: 1.6 g**

Pork Chops Baked in Sour Cream

Nonfat sour cream works great in this casserole.

4	pork chops, ½ inch (1.3 cm) thick	4
1	egg or equivalent egg substitute, lightly beaten	1
½ C	bread crumbs made from toasted high-fiber bread	125 mL
2 T	vinegar	30 mL
1 T	sugar	15 mL
½ C	nonfat sour cream	125 mL

Wash the pork chops and trim all the visible fat. Put the egg in a saucer or low bowl. Put the bread crumbs in another saucer. Dip the chops one at a time in the egg, then the crumbs to coat both sides. In a bowl, combine the rest of the ingredients. Arrange the pork chops in the bottom of a casserole. Pour the combined ingredients as a sauce over the pork chops. Cover and bake in a preheated 350°F (180°C) oven for 1 hour.

Yield: 4 servings

Each serving contains:
**calories: 318 total fat: 16.9 g saturated fat: 5.7 g cholesterol: 127 mg
sodium: 169 mg carbohydrates: 13.6 g dietary fiber: 0.7 g**

Pork Chops with Apples

Serve with a baked potato and a cooked vegetable.

6	lean pork chops	6
1 T	butter or margarine	15 mL
2	cooking apples, unpeeled, cored, and sliced ½ in. (1.25 cm) thick	2
6	maraschino cherries	6
3 T	brown sugar	45 mL

In a nonstick frying pan, over high heat, brown the pork chops on both sides. Put aside the frying pan for later use. Arrange the chops in a shallow baking dish one layer deep. Melt the butter in the frying pan that has been set aside, add the apple slices, and carefully sauté until tender. Remove the apple rings from the frying pan and put one on top of each chop. Cover tightly and bake in a preheated 350°F (180°C) oven for 45-60 minutes. Remove the casserole from the oven. Place a cherry in the center of each apple ring. Sprinkle the brown sugar over all. Baste with any drippings to moisten sugar. Bake, uncovered, for another 15 minutes. The chops should not be pink in the center when cut.

Yield: 6 servings

Each serving contains:
**calories: 585 total fat: 17.3 g saturated fat: 6.4 g cholesterol: 79 mg
sodium: 201 mg carbohydrates: 85.5 g dietary fiber: 3.5 g**

Apple-Glazed Pork Roast

Use slices of cold, leftover roast for sandwiches.

2 lb.	loin of pork	900 g
½ C	apple juice	125 mL
1 T	Worcestershire sauce	15 mL
1	small apple, peeled cored and sliced	1

Trim all the visible fat from the roast. Place the meat on a rack set into a roasting pan. Mix together the apple juice and Worcestershire sauce. Pour the apple juice mixture over the meat. Cover. Roast in a preheated 350°F (180°C) oven for about 70 minutes. Continue cooking and baste with pan juices for about 30 minutes or until glazed and the meat thermometer registers "well done for pork."

Yields: 8 servings

Each serving contains:
**calories: 194 total fat: 11.2 g saturated fat: 3.9 g cholesterol: 56 mg
sodium: 66 mg carbohydrates: 4.8 g dietary fiber: 0.5 g**

Easy Steak Bake

Cranberries are the surprise ingredient. You'll agree they are not just for turkey anymore.

3 T	flour	45 mL
1 t	salt	5 mL
2 lb.	round steak, cut ½ in. (1.25 cm) thick	900 g
2 T	canola oil	30 mL
¼ C	lemon juice	60 mL
½ t	Worcestershire sauce	3 mL
½ C	water	125 mL
1 lb.	whole cranberry sauce	450 g
½ C	chopped celery	125 mL
1 T	sugar	15 mL

Stir the flour and salt together and spread onto a plate that is about the same size as the steak. Turn the steak over and over on the plate so that the flour adheres to the meat. Heat the oil in a skillet, add the meat, and brown it on both sides. In a bowl, combine the lemon juice, Worcestershire sauce, and water. Pour the mixture over the steak. Cover and simmer for 45 minutes. Spoon the cranberry sauce, celery, and sugar over the steak. Cover and simmer for an additional hour until the meat is tender.

Yield: 8 servings

Each serving contains:

**calories: 305 total fat: 17.2 g saturated fat: 5.6 g cholesterol: 67 mg
sodium: 497 mg carbohydrates: 14.8 g dietary fiber: 2.5 g**

Old-Fashioned Beef Stew

Usually served over mashed potatoes.

2 T	flour	30 mL
grind	black pepper	grind
1 lb.	lean beef, cut into cubes	450 g
2 T	safflower oil	30 mL
1 T	wine vinegar	15 mL
2	bay leaves	2
½ t	onion powder	3 mL
½ t	garlic powder	3 mL
1 t	tomato paste	5 mL
½ t	basil	3 mL
3 C	hot water	750 mL
½ C	vermouth	125 mL
4	medium potatoes, cut into chunks	4
2	carrots, peeled and cut into chunks	2
4	medium onions, peeled and quartered	4

In a paper bag, shake the flour and pepper with cubes of meat to coat lightly with flour. Heat the oil in a Dutch oven or casserole. Brown the meat in the oil, turning frequently. Add all the seasonings, water, and vermouth and stir to mix. Heat just to the boiling point. Turn down heat, cover and simmer for 1¼ hours, or until almost done. Add the potatoes, carrots, and onions and stir; cover and simmer for 40 minutes until the potatoes are cooked.

Yield: 4 servings

Each serving contains:
**calories: 415 total fat: 12.8 g saturated fat: 2.6 g cholesterol: 66 mg
sodium: 643 mg carbohydrates: 36 g dietary fiber: 5.1 g**

Beef and Vegetable Kebobs

Perfect for outdoor grilling.

1½ lb.	trimmed beef cut into 1-1½ inch (2.5-4 cm) cubes	675 g
⅓ C	soy sauce	80 mL
⅓ C	sherry wine	80 mL
2 T	sugar	30 mL
2 T	garlic, minced fine	30 mL
12	small white onions	12
12	large mushrooms, washed and dried	12
3	large green peppers, seeded, and cut into 1 inch(2.5 cm) square	3

Place the beef in a shallow non-metallic bowl. In another bowl, mix together the soy sauce, sherry, sugar, and garlic. Pour this mixture over the beef. Stir. Cover and refrigerate for eight hours or more. In a small saucepan, bring enough water to a boil to accommodate the onions. Drop the onions into the boiling water and parboil for 3-5 minutes to tenderize and so the skins will slip off easily. Slip off skins after running cool water over the onions. Make the kebobs by alternating the beef chunks, onions, mushrooms, and green pepper pieces on 10 inch (25 cm) skewers. (If you are using wooden skewers, soak them for an hour or so before use). Grill the kebobs, basting with the remainder of the soy mixture.

Yield: 12 kebobs

Each kebob contains:
calories: 137 total fat: 3.0 g saturated fat: 1.0 g cholesterol: 33 mg sodium: 951 mg carbohydrates: 11.3 g dietary fiber: 2.6 g

Beef and Noodles in Lemon Sauce

A fresh taste. You'll want to make this recipe again and again.

1 C	fine egg noodles	250 mL
2 T	butter or margarine	30 mL
¾ C	onions, diced	185 mL
1½ lb.	leanest ground beef	675 g
1 lb.	mushrooms, sliced	450 g
¾ C	water	185 mL
2	egg yolks	2
3 T	lemon juice (fresh is best)	45 mL
2 T	sherry	30 mL

Put the noodles into a heat-resistant mixing bowl and cover them with boiling water. Set aside for 20 minutes, then drain. In a frying pan, melt the butter, add the onions, and sauté five minutes or so. Add the beef, mushrooms, and noodles. Increase heat to high and cook for another five minutes, stirring constantly. Add the water and cook another ten minutes over low heat. In a small bowl, mix together the egg yolks, lemon juice, and sherry. Scoop a few spoonfuls of the meat mixture into the bowl of egg mixture. Turn the contents of the bowl into the skillet. Heat gently while stirring. Serve over the noodles.

Yield: 6 servings

Each serving contains:
**calories: 264 total fat: 11.7 g saturated fat: 4.9 g cholesterol: 153 mg
sodium: 185 mg carbohydrates: 9.8 g dietary fiber: 1.4 g**

Meat Loaf

In this recipe, turkey stands in for half the beef.

1 lb.	ground turkey (be sure it's lean)	450 g
1 lb.	lean ground beef	450 g
2	eggs or equivalent egg substitute	2
1	onion, diced fine	1
1 C	bread crumbs	250 mL
1 T	steak sauce	15 mL

Mix all the ingredients together until well blended. Fold into a loaf pan. Bake in a preheated 350°F (180°C) oven for 45 to 50 minutes. When you remove the loaf from the oven, pour out any liquid fat. Cool slightly before cutting.

Yield: 8 servings

Each serving contains:

calories: 222 total fat: 5.8 g saturated fat: 1.8 g cholesterol: 120 mg sodium: 278 mg carbohydrates: 11.1 g dietary fiber: 1.0 g

Meat Squares

An excellent version of meat loaf for anyone on a low-acid diet or anyone who loves good food.

1 lb.	lean ground beef	450 g
1 lb.	lean ground turkey	450 g
1 C	bread crumbs	250 mL
1½ C	apples, pealed, cored, and chopped	375 mL
½ C	onion, diced	125 mL
2 T	fresh parsley, chopped	30 mL
½ t	basil	3 mL
½ t	oregano	3 mL
2	eggs, or equivalent egg substitute, lightly beaten	2

In a mixing bowl, combine all the ingredients. Spoon the mixture into an 8 inch (30 cm) pan coated with a nonstick cooking spray. Bake in a preheated 350°F (180°C) oven for 1 hour.

Yield: 9 squares

Each square contains:
calories: 208 total fat: 5.3 g saturated fat: 1.6 g cholesterol: 107 mg sodium: 195 mg carbohydrates: 12.7 g dietary fiber: 1.3 g

Hamburger Stroganoff

This is a low-calorie Americanized version of the old-country favorite. Serve over noodles.

1 lb.	ground beef, the leaner the better	450 g
1 T	butter or margarine	15 mL
½ C	minced onion	125 mL
2 T	flour	30 mL
½ C	sliced mushrooms, fresh or canned (optional)	125 mL
1 can	low-fat cream of chicken soup	1 can
1 C	fat-free sour cream	250 mL
2 T	parsley, minced	30 mL

Heat a frying pan. Add the ground beef and stir constantly to brown. Pour off any fat and discard it. Turn the browned hamburger into a bowl and set it aside. Heat the butter in a frying pan, add the onion and sauté until it is soft. Sprinkle the flour over the onion. Stir. Add the soup, mushrooms, if desired, and simmer uncovered, stirring for 10 minutes. Add the hamburger and sour cream. Heat a moment or two. Sprinkle with parsley.

Yield: 4 servings

Each serving contains:
calories: 480 total fat: 35 g saturated fat: 14.8 g cholesterol: 108 mg sodium: 714* mg carbohydrates: 11.3 g dietary fiber: 1.0 g
*Using homemade chicken soup can reduce the sodium level significantly.

Swedish Meatballs

Baking the meatballs makes them much faster to prepare.

1 lb.	very lean ground beef	450 g
1	egg or equivalent egg substitute	1
1	small onion, grated or minced	1
3 slices	high-fiber bread ground into 1 C (250 mL) crumbs	3 slices
¾ t	allspice	4 mL
1 t	sugar	5 mL
dash	white pepper	dash
¼ t	nutmeg	2 mL

Mix all the ingredients lightly and form them into small meatballs, using one tablespoon (15 mL) per meatball. Put them on a broiler pan (so the fat will drip down and away from the meat). Bake in a 375°F (190°C) oven for approximately 12 to 15 minutes.

Yield: 32 meatballs

Each meatball contains:
  **calories: 30 total fat: 0.9 g saturated fat: 0.3 g cholesterol: 150 mg
  sodium: 408 mg carbohydrates: 1.5 g dietary fiber: 0.1 g**

Jumbo Stuffed Mushrooms

Serve with brown rice and a cooked vegetable for a hearty meal.

24	large fresh mushrooms (about 2 in., or 5 cm)	24
1 lb.	lean ground beef	450 g
1	egg or equivalent egg substitute, beaten lightly	1
3 T	cold water	45 mL
½ t	lemon juice	3 mL
1 t	Worcestershire sauce	5 mL

| 1 | medium onion, grated | 1 |
| ½ C | beef stock or beef bouillon | 125 mL |

Wash and pat dry mushrooms. Remove the stems and chop them up. Mix together the mushroom stems, ground beef, egg, water, lemon juice, Worcestershire sauce, onion, and beef stock. Place the mushroom caps, hollow-side up, in a shallow baking pan coated with non-stick cooking spray. Spoon the hamburger mixture into mushroom caps. Bake in a preheated 350°F (180°C) oven 30 minutes or more until the hamburger mixture is thoroughly cooked.

Yield: 24 stuffed mushroom caps

Each mushroom cap contains:
  **calories: 68 total fat: 5.3 g saturated fat: 2.1 g cholesterol: 25 mg
  sodium: 70 mg carbohydrates: 1.2 g dietary fiber: 0.3 g**

Turkey Surprise

Use leftover turkey and serve over toast or with rice or noodles.

2 T	butter or margarine	30 mL
¼ C	onion, diced	60 mL
4 T	flour	60 mL
2 C	chicken broth	500 mL
1 T	Worcestershire sauce	15 mL
3 C	leftover, cooked turkey, diced	750 mL

Melt the butter in a saucepan. Add the onion and sauté gently until soft. Stir in the flour and cook the two gently until the flour mixture becomes bubbly. Add the rest of the ingredients and cook until thickened, about 20 minutes.

Yield: 6 servings

Each serving contains:
  **calories: 231 total fat: 12.2 g saturated fat: 4.7 g cholesterol: 75 mg
  sodium: 674 mg carbohydrates: 5.3 g dietary fiber: 0.1 g**

Easy Turkey Shepherd's Pie

Be sure you buy lean ground turkey. Some have more fat than fatty hamburger!

¾ lb.	lean ground turkey	340 g
1 (10¾ oz.) can	condensed low-fat cream of chicken soup	1 (290 g) can
1 C	skim milk	250 mL
1 T	cornstarch	15 mL
1 C	frozen peas	250 mL
1 C	frozen green beans	250 mL
2 C	cooked potatoes, mashed without butter or margarine	500 mL

Heat a nonstick frying pan and add the turkey. Cook, stirring until meat is no longer pink, about five minutes. In a bowl, combine the soup, milk, and cornstarch. Stir into the turkey and cook until the mixture begins to boil. Add the peas and green beans. Combine and spoon into four individual-serving ovenproof casserole dishes. Top each one with one-quarter of the mashed potatoes. Bake in a pre-heated 400°F (200°C) oven for 15-20 minutes, until the potatoes are lightly browned. (You can use a single, larger casserole dish, but cooking will take less time. Watch the potatoes after 10 minutes. Adjust the time in the oven.)

Yield: 4 servings

Each serving contains:
**calories: 244 total fat: 4.2 g saturated fat: 1.5 g cholesterol: 57 mg
sodium: 684 mg carbohydrates: 19.4 g dietary fiber: 4.0 g**

Baked Chicken Salad

Use up leftover chicken or start by cooking boneless breasts in water.

1 C	fat-free mayonnaise	250 mL
2 C	cooked chicken, without skin, cubed	500 mL

2 C	celery, sliced thinly	500 mL
1 C	toasted bread, cubed	250 mL
¼ C	slivered almonds, toasted	125 mL
2 T	lemon juice	30 mL
2 t	onion, grated	10 mL
½ C	Cheddar cheese, diced	125 mL
⅓ C	fat-free potato chips, crushed	80 mL

Combine the mayonnaise, chicken, celery, bread cubes, almonds, lemon juice, and onion in a large bowl. Spoon the mixture into six individual serving dishes that have been coated with nonstick cooking spray. Top with cheese and crushed potato chips. Bake in a preheated 450°F (230°C) oven 10 to 15 minutes.

Yield: 4 servings

Each serving contains:
**calories: 415 total fat: 14.4 g saturated fat: 4.6 g cholesterol: 79 mg
sodium: 821 mg carbohydrates: 42.1 g dietary fiber: 3.2 g**

Chicken Salad

Fat-free mayonnaise puts this summer favorite back on the menu for anyone on a heartburn-decreasing diet.

2 C	cubed, cold cooked chicken	500 mL
1 C	diced celery	250 mL
1 T	lemon juice	15 mL
½ C	fat-free mayonnaise	125 mL
3	hard boiled diced eggs	3

Mix together the chicken, celery, and lemon juice. Stir in the mayonnaise to coat. Fold in the eggs carefully. Chill before serving.

Yield: 6 servings

Each serving contains:
**calories: 160 total fat: 6.7 g saturated fat: 1.9 g cholesterol: 158 mg
sodium: 191 mg carbohydrates: 4.3 g dietary fiber: 0.4 g**

Chinese Almond Chicken

This tastes great over hot cooked rice!

1 T	canola oil	15 mL
2 C	chicken, cooked and diced	500 mL
2 C	celery, sliced	500 mL
½ C	mushrooms, sliced	125 mL
½ C	bamboo shoots, sliced thin	125 mL
1 C	snow pea pods	250 mL
2 T	cornstarch	30 mL
2 C	chicken broth	500 mL
1 t	low salt soy sauce	5 mL
½ C	toasted almonds	125 mL

Heat the canola oil in a frying pan. Add the chicken and sauté while stirring constantly until the chicken is lightly browned. Add the celery, mushrooms, bamboo shoots, and peas and stir the mixture. Sauté for an additional 5 minutes, then set aside. Put the cornstarch in a saucepan and, over medium heat, gradually add the chicken broth. Cook, stirring constantly, until the mixture thickens and comes to a boil. Stir in the soy sauce. Add the chicken-vegetable mixture. Simmer, covered, for an additional 5 minutes. Sprinkle with toasted almonds.

Yield: 6 servings

Each serving contains:

**calories: 248 total fat: 13.7 g saturated fat: 2.2 g cholesterol: 44 mg
sodium: 687 mg carbohydrates: 10.5 g dietary fiber: 3.1 g**

Chicken "Scallopini"

Yes, scalloppini without tomatoes is possible and so delicious you won't miss them.

2 T	flour	30 mL
dash	freshly ground pepper (optional)	dash
2 (½ lb.)	boneless, skinless chicken breasts	2 (225 g)
2 t	olive oil	10 mL
2 T	minced onions	30 mL
⅓ C	apricot nectar	80 mL
⅓ C	fat-free chicken broth	80 mL
1 T	cider vinegar	15 mL
1 t	brown sugar	5 mL
3	dried apricot halves, chopped	3

Sprinkle the flour over a dinner plate. Add pepper, if desired. Stir. Wet the chicken breasts under cold running water and place them on top of the flour. Press down to coat. Turn the chicken over to coat the other side. Heat the oil in a medium-sized skillet. Add the chicken and cook 3 or 4 minutes on each side. The outside will be golden brown. The inside will no longer be pink. Remove the cooked chicken to a clean plate. Cover to keep warm. Add the minced onion to the remaining oil in the pan. Stir well and cook for a minute or so. Add the rest of the ingredients, stir, and bring to a boil. Cook for 4 or 5 minutes, until the apricot pieces are tender. Spoon the sauce over the chicken breasts. Serve immediately.

Yield: 2 servings

Each serving contains:
  **calories: 239 total fat: 6.1 g saturated fat: 1.0 g cholesterol: 65 mg
  sodium: 160 mg carbohydrates: 17.4 g dietary fiber: 1.0 g**

Chicken à la King

Serve over noodles or rice.

1½ T	butter or margarine	22 mL
3 T	flour	45 mL
1½ C	low-fat chicken broth	375 mL
1 C	cooked chicken, diced	250 mL
½ C	mushrooms, sautéed	125 mL
1	egg yolk	1
1 t	dry sherry, if desired	5 mL

Melt the butter in a saucepan. Add the flour and cook, stirring for a few minutes. Gradually add the chicken broth and cook until the sauce is smooth and boiling. Add the chicken and mushrooms. Remove from heat. Put the egg yolk into a small bowl. Spoon a few scoops of the sauce over the egg yolk. Combine. Add the egg yolk mixture to the saucepan. Stir and cook a few minutes until it thickens slightly. Add the sherry, if desired.

Yield: 4 servings

Each serving contains:
  **calories: 158 total fat: 8.8 g saturated fat: 3.9 g cholesterol: 97 mg
  sodium: 185 mg carbohydrates: 5.9 g dietary fiber: 0.1 g**

Quick Chicken Noodle Casserole

Just like Mother used to make, but low in fat.

3 C	uncooked egg noodles (wide are best)	750 mL
2 T	water	30 mL
2 halves		2 halves
(10 oz.)	chicken breast, in ½ in. (1.2 cm) cubes	(30 g)
1	onion, diced	1
10¾ oz.		290 g
1 can	low-fat condensed cream of chicken soup	1 can
1 C	nonfat milk	250 mL
3 C	frozen cut-up broccoli	750 mL

Cook the noodles in boiling water according to the package directions. Drain them and set aside. Meanwhile, heat the 2 T (30 mL) of water in a nonstick frying pan. Add the chicken and onion. Cook and stir until the chicken is cooked through. (It will no longer be pink inside). Stir in the soup and milk. Cook until the mixture begins to bubble. Add the broccoli and noodles. Cook until the mixture is thoroughly heated.

Yield: 6 servings

Each serving contains:
**calories: 220 total fat: 7.2 g saturated fat: 2.2 g cholesterol: 53 mg
sodium: 554 mg carbohydrates: 19.2 g dietary fiber: 2.6 g**

Chicken Marsala

If the small amount of wine in this recipe bothers your stomach, substitute low-fat chicken broth and sherry flavoring for the Marsala.

¼ C	flour	60 mL
dash	white pepper	dash
dash	oregano	dash
dash	basil	dash
1¼ lb.	boneless, skinless chicken breasts	600 g
1 T	safflower oil	15 mL
1 T	butter or margarine	15 mL
½ lb.	mushrooms, sliced	225 g
1 C	Marsala wine or dry sherry	250 mL

Mix the flour, white pepper, oregano, and basil together on a plate. Wash and dry the chicken breasts and coat each with the flour mixture. Reserve any leftover flour. Heat the oil and butter in a frying pan. Add the chicken breasts and sauté gently until brown and tender on both sides, about 15 minutes. Remove the breasts to a dish. Add the mushrooms and ¼ cup (60 mL) of the wine; cook for about 5 minutes over low heat. Scrape the bottom of the pan to loosen any flour. Stir in any reserved flour and the remaining wine. Simmer until the mixture thickens, stirring constantly. Slip the cooked breasts into the sauce. Cook gently for about 5 minutes or more.

Yield: 4 servings

Each serving contains:
**calories: 333 total fat: 17.1 g saturated fat: 5.1 g cholesterol: 80 mg
sodium: 106 mg carbohydrates: 9.1 g dietary fiber: 0.7 g**

Chicken Fricassee

A classic recipe that is so easy to fix, it almost cooks by itself.
Traditionally served with biscuits and mashed potatoes.

4 (2 lb.)	chicken breasts, trimmed	4 (900 g)
¼ C	flour	60 mL
½ t	white pepper	3 mL
2 T	safflower oil	30 mL
1	medium onion, diced fine	1
1	clove garlic, minced	1
2 C	water	500 mL
2 T	cornstarch	30 mL
⅓ C	fresh parsley, chopped	80 mL

Wash and skin the chicken. Remove any visible fat. Mix the flour and pepper together on a plate. Coat each piece of chicken by rolling it in the flour mixture. Heat the oil in a large saucepan or Dutch oven. Add the onion and garlic; cook gently for 2 to 3 minutes; add the chicken and cook for a few minutes on each side until golden brown. Add the water; cover the pot tightly and gently simmer for about 45 minutes, or until tender; remove the chicken to a plate.

Measure the cornstarch into a bowl. Gradually stir in a cup of the cooking liquid and pour it back into the cooking pot. Heat and stir until the sauce thickens. Stir in the parsley. Reheat the chicken in the sauce.

Yield: 4 servings

Each serving contains:
calories: 326 total fat: 9.4 g saturated fat: 1.2 g cholesterol: 105 mg
sodium: 275 mg carbohydrates: 14.1 g dietary fiber: 1.1 g

Chicken with Melon

A lovely presentation for a warm evening.

2 C	fat-free chicken broth	500 mL
2	celery ribs, diced	2
2	carrots, peeled and diced	2
4	boneless, skinless chicken breasts	4
1	large honeydew melon	1

Bring the chicken broth to a boil in a saucepan. Add the celery, carrots, and chicken breasts and poach, covered, over low heat for 20 minutes or so, until the chicken breasts are cooked through. Remove the chicken from the liquid and chill the chicken. (Cook some rice in the leftover broth and vegetables and make soup; you won't need the broth again for this recipe.) Slice half the melon into six wedges. Discard the seeds. Save the scraps and wedges. Make as many melon balls as possible from the other half. Chill the melon balls and scraps of melon. Before serving, place one wedge on each dinner plate, and divide the melon scraps next to the wedges. Using a scissors, cut the chicken into bite-sized pieces. Mix the melon balls and chicken together. Spoon over the wedges.

Yield: 6 servings

Each serving contains:
**calories: 259 total fat: 9.2 g saturated fat: 2.6 g cholesterol: 62 mg
sodium: 198 mg carbohydrates: 23 g dietary fiber: 2.2 g**

Chow Mein

Check the fat content on canned chow mein. You'll find it's worth it to make your own from scratch.

1	medium onion	1
½	green pepper	½
6	medium mushrooms	6

1 C	mung sprouts	250 mL
10 oz.	boneless chicken breasts	280 g
3 T	lemon juice	45 mL
1 T	sugar	15 mL
3 T	sherry	45 mL
⅔ C	boiling water	170 mL
1 T	peanut oil	15 mL
1	clove garlic, peeled	1
2 T	cornstarch	30 mL

Prepare the vegetables: Cut the onion and green pepper into chunks; slice the mushrooms and sprouts; and arrange the vegetables on a plate. Cut the chicken into thin strips and put them on a plate so they are ready for frying. Combine 2 tablespoons (30 mL) of the lemon juice, the sugar and 2 tablespoons (30 mL) of sherry in a small bowl. Stir in the boiling water; set aside. Heat the oil in a wok or skillet over a medium heat. Add the garlic for a minute or so until you can smell it. Add the onions and stir-fry for 30 seconds (push the onion pieces from side to side with a wooden spoon, wok utensil, or spatula). Add the green pepper and stir-fry for another 30 seconds. Add the chicken and stir-fry for approximately two minutes. If you use leftover chicken breasts, this recipe is even faster. Cooked leftover pieces of meat need only be stirred in for a few seconds to heat. Add the mushrooms and stir-fry for another minute. Add the sprouts and lemon juice mixture. Stir to combine. Turn the heat down, cover and cook for three minutes. While the mixture is cooking, combine the cornstarch with remaining lemon juice and sherry. Add this to the wok and stir for another minute or two, until the sauce has thickened.

Yield: 4 servings

Each serving contains:
**calories: 196 total fat: 8.9 g saturated fat: 2.1 g cholesterol: 36 mg
sodium: 178 mg carbohydrates: 13.3 g dietary fiber: 1.6 g**

Chicken Dinner in a Pot

Nothing could be easier.

4	boneless chicken breasts, skin removed	4
4	medium potatoes, peeled, cut into ½ in (1.3 cm) slices	4
1 C	carrots, peeled and chopped into ½ in. (1.3 cm) slices	250 mL
1 C	frozen peas	250 mL
½ C	parsley, finely chopped	125 mL
¼ C	lemon juice	60 mL
¼ C	water	60 mL

Coat a baking dish that has a tight-fitting cover with a nonstick cooking spray. Place the chicken breasts in the baking dish. Top with all the rest of the ingredients and cover tightly. Bake in a preheated 375°F (190°C) oven for an hour to 1¼ hours, until the vegetables are tender. Add another quarter to half cup (60-125 mL) water if the chicken and vegetables seem to be getting dry during cooking.

Yield: 4 servings

Each serving contains:
calories: 441 total fat: 3.5 g saturated fat: 0.8 g cholesterol: 130 mg sodium: 207 mg carbohydrates: 35.9 g dietary fiber: 6.1 g

Egg Foo Yung

If you are using fresh mung bean sprouts, steam them a minute or two to soften them up.

4	eggs, or equivalent egg substitute, beaten	4
1 lb.	bean sprouts, drained	450 g
½ C	cooked chicken, diced fine	125 mL

1	small onion, diced fine	1
1 T	low-sodium soy sauce (optional)	15 mL
2 T	canola oil	30 mL

Combine eggs, bean sprouts, chicken, onion, and soy sauce, if desired. Put a small amount of oil into a frying pan. Drop a spoonful of the egg mixture into the frying pan. Cook until brown, then flip and brown the other side. Continue until all the batter is cooked, adding more oil to the frying pan, if needed. Keep the cooked patties warm while you are frying the rest.

Yield: 10 patties

Each patty contains:
**calories: 85 total fat: 5.5 g saturated fat: 1.0 g cholesterol: 91 mg
sodium: 89 mg carbohydrates: 3.6 g dietary fiber: 1.0 g**

Low-Fat Egg Salad Sandwich

Egg salad is fine with fewer yolks and fat-free mayonnaise on whole wheat bread.

4	eggs, hard boiled	4
2	sweet gherkin pickles, diced	2
¼ C	fat-free mayonnaise	60 mL
6	slices, whole wheat or high-fiber bread	6
3	leaves of lettuce, washed and dried	3

Peel the eggs and throw away two yolks (optional). Dice the remaining eggs fine. Combine them in a mixing bowl with the pickles and mayonnaise. Mix well. Spread one-third of the egg salad on each of 3 slices of bread. Cover each with a lettuce leaf and the second slice of bread.

Yield: 3 sandwiches

Each sandwich contains:
**calories: 360 total fat: 10 g saturated fat: 2.7 g cholesterol: 292 mg
sodium: 595 mg carbohydrates: 50 g dietary fiber: 11.5 g**

Juneau Omelet

The first time I had this was in Fiddlehead restaurant in Juneau, Alaska. This is the low-fat version.

4	eggs or equivalent egg substitute, beaten	4
¼ C	fat-free sour cream	60 mL
2 t	minced onion	10 mL
3 oz.	fat-free cream cheese cut into ½ inch (1.3 cm) cubes	85 g

Heat a frying pan. Coat with a nonstick cooking spray. Pour in the beaten eggs slowly while moving the pan to coat evenly. As the egg cooks and thickens at the edges, lift the edges with a spatula or rubber scraper and tilt the pan so the uncooked egg flows underneath. When the bottom is lightly brown and the top is mostly thickened spread the sour cream over the top. Then sprinkle on the onion and the cut-up cream cheese cubes. Carefully fold one-half the omelet over the other. Lower the heat for a minute or two so that the cream cheese will soften.

Yield: 3 servings

Each serving contains:
calories: 138 total fat: 6.7 g saturated fat: 2.1 g cholesterol: 288 mg sodium: 244 mg carbohydrates: 4.9 g dietary fiber: 0 g

Broccoli-Egg Bake

Try this casserole with homemade soup and bread for a cozy Sunday night supper.

10 oz. pkg.	frozen broccoli	284 g pkg.
2 T	butter or margarine	30 mL
2 T	flour	30 mL
1 C	fat-free milk	250 mL
½ C	low-fat American cheese, shredded	125 mL
6	eggs, hard-boiled, shelled and sliced	6

Cook the broccoli according to package directions. Drain. Set aside. In a small saucepan, melt the butter and blend in the flour. Slowly add the milk and cook, stirring constantly until sauce thickens, about 3-5 minutes. Add the cheese and stir until it melts. Arrange 2 layers of broccoli and eggs in sauce in a small casserole that has been coated with a nonstick cooking spray. Pour the sauce evenly over the casserole. Bake in a preheated oven 350°F (180°C) oven for 30 minutes.

Yield: 4 servings

Each serving contains:
calories: 236 total fat: 13.6 g saturated fat: 6.0 g cholesterol: 338 mg sodium: 391 mg carbohydrates: 12.5 g dietary fiber: 2.1 g

Chapter 6
BREADS AND MUFFINS

German Blueberry Kuchen

Great for breakfast or dessert. Serve warm.

1½ C	sifted flour	375 mL
2 t	baking powder	10 mL
¾ C	sugar	185 mL
¼ C	butter or margarine, softened	60 mL
⅔ C	nonfat milk	170 mL
1 t	vanilla	5 mL
1	egg or equivalent egg substitute	1
1 C	blueberries (fresh or thawed frozen)	250 mL
3 T	sugar	45 mL

Sift the flour with the baking powder and sugar. In another bowl, mix together the butter, milk, and vanilla. Combine these wet and dry ingredients and mix with an electric mixer for at least three minutes. Add the egg and beat again for two minutes. Transfer to an 8 inch (20 cm) square pan that has been coated with a nonstick cooking spray. Mix the blueberries and the 3 T (45 mL) of sugar together. Put this mixture on top of the batter. Bake in a preheated 350°F (180°C) oven for 40-45 minutes. The top will be lightly browned. Cut into 9 squares.

Yield: 9 squares

Each square contains:
**calories: 226 total fat: 5.9 g saturated fat: 3.4 g cholesterol: 38 mg
sodium: 150 mg carbohydrates: 40.2 g dietary fiber: 0.4 g**

Quick Oatmeal Bread

This bread only rises once. It has a wonderful homemade flavor.

½ C	boiling water	125 mL
¼ C	skim milk	60 mL
½ C	"old-fashioned" oatmeal, not quick or instant oats	125 mL
3 T	safflower oil	45 mL
¼ C	molasses	60 mL
¼ C	warm water	60 mL
pinch	sugar	pinch
1 T	active dry yeast	15 mL
1	egg or equivalent egg substitute	1
2¾ C	flour	685 mL

Stir together the boiling water, milk, oatmeal, oil and molasses in a mixing bowl. Cool until lukewarm. Meanwhile, put the ¼ cup (60 mL) warm water into a small bowl. Add the pinch of sugar and stir in the yeast. Let sit for 2 to 5 minutes. Add the yeast to the oatmeal mixture. Stir in the egg and about half the flour. Beat for 3 or 4 minutes with an electric mixer, adding the remaining flour gradually. Mix until the flour is blended in and the batter smooth; it will still be sticky. Scrape the dough into a loaf pan sprayed with nonstick spray. Smooth it into the corners. Cover the pan with a cloth and set it in a warm place. Let it rise only to the top of the pan. While the dough is rising, preheat the oven to 375°F (190°C). Bake for about 50 to 55 minutes.

Yield: 20 slices

Each slice contains:
**calories: 106 total fat: 2.7 g saturated fat: 0.3 g cholesterol: 11 mg
sodium: 28 mg carbohydrates: 17.7 g dietary fiber: 0.4 g**

Quick Bran Rolls

Wonderful warmed for breakfast, and they freeze well.

⅓ C	sugar	80 mL
½ C	bran	125 mL
½ C	safflower oil	125 mL
½ C	boiling water	125 mL
½ C	warm water	125 mL
pinch	sugar	pinch
1 T	active dry yeast	15 mL
1	egg or equivalent egg substitute	1
3 C	flour	750 mL

Combine the sugar, bran, oil, and boiling water in a large mixing bowl; stir and cool to lukewarm. In a small bowl combine the warm water, pinch of sugar, and yeast; stir. Let stand for 2 to 5 minutes. Add the egg to the lukewarm bran mixture and stir well. Mix in the yeast mixture. Gradually stir in the flour. Mix until the flour is blended in and the batter is smooth. Cover the bowl with a cloth and set it in a warm place for two hours or so, until double. Stir the batter and put it into 24 muffin pan cups sprayed with a nonstick spray, filling them up about halfway. Cover the pans with the cloth and set it in a warm place. Let it rise *only* to the top of the pan. While the dough is rising, preheat oven to 375°F (190°C). Bake for about 50 to 55 minutes.

Yield: 20 rolls

Each roll contains:
**calories: 138 total fat: 6.0 g saturated fat: 0.6 g cholesterol: 11 mg
sodium: 4 mg carbohydrates: 18.9 g dietary fiber: 0.8 g**

Cape Cod Bread

Make this in the morning and let it rise while you are at work. Or, make the dough at night and bake it in the morning.

1 T	yeast	15 mL
⅓ C	warm water	80 mL
pinch	sugar	pinch
4 C	flour	1 L
1 t	salt	5 mL
1 C	sugar	250 mL
4	eggs or equivalent egg substitute, lightly beaten	4
⅔ C	nonfat milk, heated to lukewarm	170 mL
⅓ C	butter or margarine, melted	80 mL

Put yeast in a cup or small bowl. Add the warm water and a pinch of sugar. Stir and then set aside. In a large bowl, sift the flour and salt together. In another bowl, mix the sugar, eggs, and milk together. Add the flour mixture and the yeast. Knead on a lightly floured board until the dough is smooth and yielding. This may take up to 10 minutes. Add the melted butter and knead again. Return dough to the bowl, cover with a tea towel, set in a warm place, and let rise until doubled in bulk (often 12 hours). Divide the dough into 3 slightly flat loaves. Roll the dough in flour and place each loaf in a pie plate that has been coated with a nonstick cooking spray. Bake in a pre-heated 350°F (180°C) oven for 40-50 minutes, or until the loaves are golden-brown.

Yield: 3 loaves of bread; 22 slices per loaf

Each slice contains:
calories: 53 total fat: 1.3 g saturated fat: 0.7 g cholesterol: 15 mg sodium: 47 mg carbohydrates: 9 g dietary fiber: 0.1 g

Pumpkin Biscuits

These bake up on cookie sheets and have a rich flavor.

2 C	flour, sifted	500 mL
3 T	sugar	45 mL
4 t	baking powder	20 mL
4 T	butter or margarine	60 mL
4 T	fat-free cream cheese	60 mL
⅓ C	pecans, chopped(optional)	80 mL
¾ C	nonfat sour cream	185 mL
⅔ C	canned pumpkin	170 mL

Sift together the flour, sugar, and baking powder. Using two knives or a pastry cutter, cut in the butter and cream cheese and blend until the mixture looks like course meal or crumbs. Add the pecans, if desired. In another bowl combine the sour cream and the pumpkin. Sir the pumpkin mixture into the flour mixture. Don't overmix; stir just enough to moisten. The dough will be stiff. Knead it a few times. Dust a breadboard with a little flour. Roll out the dough to a thickness of ½ inch (1.3 cm) and use a teacup or a biscuit cutter to cut circular biscuits. Place the biscuits on a cookie sheet coated with a nonstick cooking spray. Leave an inch (2.5 cm) between each biscuit. Bake in a preheated 450°F (230°C) oven for 20 minutes. They will be golden-brown. Serve at once.

Yield: 20 biscuits

Each biscuit contains:
**calories: 83 total fat: 2.4 g saturated fat: 1.4 g cholesterol: 7 mg
sodium: 117 mg carbohydrates: 13 g dietary fiber: 0.1 g**

Banana Tea Loaf

The fat-free sour cream lowers the fat and the calories. Serve as dessert or as a dinner bread with a light meal.

1¾ C	flour, sifted	435 mL
¾ t	baking soda	4 mL
1¼ t	cream of tartar	7 mL
2	eggs or equivalent egg substitute	2
¼ C	soft butter or margarine	60 mL
¼ C	fat-free sour cream	60 mL
2	ripe bananas, mashed	2
¾ C	sugar	185 mL

Sift the flour, baking soda, and cream of tartar together into a mixing bowl. Place the eggs, butter, sour cream, bananas and sugar into a blender or food processor and blend until smooth. Pour this wet mixture over the dry ingredients and combine gently just until moist. Transfer to a loaf pan prepared with a nonstick cooking spray. Bake in a preheated 350°F (180°C) oven for 45 minutes.

Yield: 16 slices

Each slice contains:
**calories: 137 total fat: 3.7 g saturated fat: 2.0 g cholesterol: 34 mg
sodium: 58 mg carbohydrates: 24 g dietary fiber: 0.3 g**

Texas Spoon Bread

Try this with a casserole or barbecue meal.

1 C	cornmeal	250 mL
3 C	nonfat milk	750 mL
3	eggs or equivalent egg substitute, well beaten	3
1 t	salt (optional)	5 mL
1 T	baking powder	15 mL
1 T	butter or margarine	15 mL

In a saucepan, combine the cornmeal and 2 cups (500 mL) of the milk. Bring the mixture to a boil, stirring constantly. Add the remaining milk along with the eggs, baking powder, and butter. Stir well to combine. Turn into a 1 quart (1 L) casserole that has been prepared by being coating with a nonstick cooking spray. Bake in a preheated 350°F (180°C) oven for 30 minutes or so.

Yield: 8 servings

Each serving contains:

**calories: 137 total fat: 3.8 g saturated fat: 1.6 g cholesterol: 85 mg
sodium: 222 mg carbohydrates: 18.5 g dietary fiber: 1.3 g**

Corn Bread

A traditional Southern favorite that will be appreciated with any meal.

¾ C	flour, measured after being sifted	185 mL
2½ t	baking powder	13 mL
2 T	sugar	30 mL
¾ t	salt (optional)	4 mL
1¼ C	cornmeal	310 mL
1	egg or equivalent egg substitute	1
2 T	canola oil	30 mL
1 C	nonfat milk	250 mL

Sift the flour, baking powder, sugar, and salt together into a mixing bowl. Add the cornmeal and stir until they are well combined. In another bowl, combine the egg, oil, and milk. Pour into a 9 inch (22 cm) square pan that has been coated with nonstick cooking spray. Bake in a preheated 425°F (220°C) oven for 25 minutes.

Yield: 9 squares

Each square contains:
**calories: 86 total fat: 2.5 g saturated fat: 0.3 g cholesterol: 14 mg
sodium: 69 mg carbohydrates: 14 g dietary fiber: 1.2 g**

Old-Fashioned Drop Biscuits

Traditional with beef stew and chicken fricassee, but fast to make to serve with soup.

2 C	flour, sifted before being measured	500 mL
1 T	baking powder	15 mL
2	eggs or equivalent egg substitute	2
¾ C	nonfat sour cream	185 mL

Sift the flour and baking powder together. Mix in the eggs and sour cream. The dough should be lumpy. Drop onto an ungreased baking sheet a tablespoon at a time. Bake in a preheated 400°F (200°C) oven for 15 minutes.

Yield: 12 biscuits

Each biscuit contains:
 **calories: 137 total fat: 1.2 g saturated fat: 0.3 g cholesterol: 35 mg
 sodium: 114 mg carbohydrates: 26 g dietary fiber: 0 g**

Oat Bran Muffins

Bran muffins in the supermarket or doughnut shop may have oat bran, but also have more calories, fat, and sugar than you would think. A bran muffin from a major national doughnut chain can have 122 calories, more than the same shop's Bavarian cream–filled doughnut covered with chocolate frosting! It can also have 35% more fat. This recipe makes delicious oat bran muffins—not dry and tasteless, as many homemade oat bran muffins tend to be.

1 C	flour	250 mL
1 C	oat bran	250 mL
2 t	baking powder	10 mL
2 t	cinnamon	10 mL
½ C	brown sugar	125 mL
½ C	carrots, shredded finely	125 mL

2	large, tart apples (*i.e.,* Granny Smiths), peeled, cored, and shredded fine	2
½ C	raisins	125 mL
1 C	chopped pecans (optional)	250 mL
¼ C	safflower oil	60 mL
½ C	low-fat milk	125 mL
2	eggs or equivalent egg substitute	2
2 t	vanilla	10 mL

Prepare muffin pans by spraying with a nonstick spray. Combine the flour, oat bran, baking powder, cinnamon, and brown sugar in a large bowl. In another bowl, combine the carrots, apples, raisins, nuts, oil, milk, eggs, and vanilla. Stir until well mixed. Pour the wet ingredients over the dry ones and stir until well blended, but don't overmix. Spoon the batter into the muffin tins until they are two-thirds full. Bake in a 375°F (190°C) oven for 15 to 20 minutes until lightly browned.

Yield: 16 muffins

Each muffin contains:
**calories: 132 total fat: 4.8 g saturated fat: 0.7 g cholesterol: 27 mg
sodium: 62 mg carbohydrates: 22.4 g dietary fiber: 2.0 g**

Apple Muffins

Substantial muffins that make soup a meal, or grab one for breakfast on the run.

¾ C	whole wheat flour	185 mL
½ C	flour	125 mL
1 C	oat bran	250 mL
⅔ C	brown sugar, packed	170 mL
1 t	baking powder	5 mL
1 t	baking soda	5 mL
¼ t	salt (optional)	2 mL
¼ t	cinnamon (optional)	2 mL
1 T	vinegar	15 mL
1 C	skim milk	250 mL
2	egg whites	2
2 T	canola oil	30 mL
¾ C	grated apple (1 small apple)	185 mL

In a large mixing bowl, combine the flours, oat bran, brown sugar, baking powder, baking soda, and, if desired, salt, and cinnamon. In another bowl, combine the vinegar and milk. Let stand a minute or two before whisking in the egg whites and canola oil. Pour the wet ingredients over the dry ones. Stir until just moist. Don't beat. Stir in the grated apple. Spray 12 muffin cups with nonstick cooking spray or line with paper cups. Fill with batter about two-thirds full. Bake in a preheated 400°F (200°C) oven for 15 to 20 minutes. The muffins will be lightly browned.

Yield: 12 muffins

Each muffin contains:

**calories: 143 total fat: 3.9 g saturated fat: 0.6 g cholesterol: 36 mg
sodium: 160 mg carbohydrates: 25.8 g dietary fiber: 1.5 g**

Corn Muffins

Muffins are easy to make. Don't use an electric mixer or you'll overbeat them.

⅔ C	cornmeal	170 mL
1¾ C	flour	435 mL
¼ C	sugar	60 mL
2 T	baking powder (shake and stir before measuring)	30 mL
1	egg or equivalent egg substitute	1
3 T	safflower oil	45 mL
½ C	nonfat milk	125 mL
½ C	water	125 mL

Prepare an 8-inch (20 cm) square pan or 12 muffin cups by spraying them with a nonstick spray or brushing lightly with safflower oil. Mix the dry ingredients together in a bowl, using a whisk. In another bowl beat the eggs; add the oil, milk, and water; mix well. Pour this wet mixture over the dry mixture and stir gently, just enough to moisten. Spoon about ¼ cup (60 mL) of batter into each muffin cup. The amount in each will depend on the size of the muffin cups but as a general rule fill the cups about ⅔ to ¾ full. Alternatively, put all the batter into a square pan. Bake in a 400°F (200°C) oven about 15 to 18 minutes.

Yield: 16 muffins

Each muffin contains:
**calories: 116 total fat: 3.4 g saturated fat: 0.4 g cholesterol: 13 mg
sodium: 147 mg carbohydrates: 19 g dietary fiber: 0.4 g**

Applesauce Muffins

Good to round out a meal any time of day!

1½ C	flour	375 mL
¼ C	sugar	60 mL
2 T	baking powder	30 mL
½ t	cinnamon	3 mL
¼ t	nutmeg	2 mL
1	egg or equivalent egg substitute	1
3 T	safflower oil	45 mL
½ C	applesauce	125 mL
¼ C	skim milk	60 mL
¼ C	water	60 mL

Prepare 12 muffin cups by coating each with a nonstick spray. Mix together the flour, sugar, baking powder, cinnamon, and nutmeg in a bowl. In another bowl, beat the egg or substitute, add the safflower oil, applesauce, milk, and water, and mix well. Pour this wet mixture over the dry mixture and stir gently, just enough to moisten. Spoon about ¼ C (60 mL) of the batter into each muffin cup, about ½ to ¾ full. Bake in a 400°F (200°C) oven for 15 to 20 minutes.

Yield: 12 muffins

Each muffin contains:
calories: 115 total fat: 4.0 g saturated fat: 0.5 g cholesterol: 18 mg sodium: 192 mg carbohydrates: 17.3 g dietary fiber: 0.1 g

Bran and Carrot Muffins

High in fiber and flavor and low in fat.

1 C	40% Bran Flakes	250 mL
¼ C	fat-free milk	60 mL
2 C	carrots, shredded fine	500 mL
2 T	brown sugar	30 mL
2 T	canola oil	30 mL
1	egg or equivalent egg substitute, slightly beaten	1
1 C	whole wheat flour	250 mL
1 t	baking powder	5 mL
½ t	baking soda	3 mL

In a large mixing bowl, combine the Bran Flakes, milk, and carrots. Add the brown sugar, oil, and egg to the carrot mixture. In another bowl, mix together the flour, baking powder, and baking soda. Carefully fold the flour mixture into the carrot mixture until just moistened. Coat 12 muffin cups with nonstick cooking spray. Bake in a preheated 400°F (200°C) oven for 20-25 minutes. Cool on wire rack before serving.

Yield: 12 muffins

Each muffin contains:
**calories: 102 total fat: 3.1 g saturated fat: 0.4 g cholesterol: 18 mg
sodium: 143 mg carbohydrates: 16.7 g dietary fiber: 1.6 g**

Whole Wheat Muffins

As good as any bakery muffins.

⅔ C	all-purpose flour, sifted before being measured	170 mL
1⅓ C	whole wheat flour	330 mL
1 t	salt (optional)	5 mL
2 t	baking powder	10 mL
2 T	molasses	30 mL
1	egg or equivalent egg substitute	1
1 C	nonfat milk	250 mL
1 T	canola oil	15 mL
¼ C	raisins, chopped	60 mL

In a mixing bowl, mix the flours, salt, and baking powder until well combined. In another bowl, mix the molasses, egg, milk, and oil. Pour the wet ingredients over the dry ingredients and combine with a few quick strokes. Sprinkle the raisins over the batter and stir the minimum strokes to mix them in. Lumps are fine. Fill 20 muffin tins that have been coated with nonstick cooking spray, about ⅔ full. Bake in a preheated 400°F (200°C) oven for 20–25 minutes.

Yield: 20 muffins

Each muffin contains:
   calories: 74 total fat: 1.5 g saturated fat: 0.2 g cholesterol: 11 mg
      sodium: 50 mg carbohydrates: 13.3 g dietary fiber: 0.1 g

Blueberry Muffins

My favorite! You can substitute frozen cranberries for the blueberries.

3 C	flour (sifted before being measured)	750 mL
½ C	sugar	125 mL
2 T	baking powder	30 mL
½ C	safflower oil	125 mL
3	eggs or equivalent egg substitute	3
½ C	skim milk	125 mL
½ C	water	125 mL
1 C	blueberries, fresh or frozen (but not defrosted)	250 mL
sprinkle	confectioners' sugar (optional)	sprinkle

Prepare the muffin tins with a nonstick spray. Sift together the flour, sugar, and baking powder in a large bowl. In another bowl combine the oil, eggs, milk, and water. Stir until well mixed. Pour the wet ingredients into the bowl of dry ingredients and stir only until blended, but don't overmix. Add the berries and stir lightly. Spoon the batter into the muffin tins until they are two-thirds full. Bake in a 400°F (200°C) oven for 15 to 18 minutes until lightly browned. Sprinkle with confectioners' sugar before serving.

Yield: 24 muffins

Each muffin contains:
**calories: 130 total fat: 5.5 g saturated fat: 0.7 g cholesterol: 27 mg
sodium: 103 mg carbohydrates: 17.6 g dietary fiber: 0.2 g**

Chapter 7
MISCELLANEOUS

Crab Quiche Canapés

Buy phyllo shells in the freezer section of the supermarket.

1	egg or equivalent egg substitute, beaten	1
½ C	fat-free milk	125 mL
½ t	Parmesan cheese, grated	3 mL
2 T	crabmeat, finely chopped	30 mL
1 pkg.	phyllo shells	1 pkg.

Combine the egg, milk, cheese, and crabmeat in a small bowl. Place one tablespoon (15 mL) of the mixture in each phyllo shell. Bake in a preheated 325°F (160°C) oven for 15 minutes or until the quiche has set. Keep the canapés hot in an electric skillet or on a hot buffet tray.

Yield: 12 canapés

Each canapé contains:
  **calories: 16 total fat: 0.6 g saturated fat: 0.2 g cholesterol: 19 mg
  sodium: 24 mg carbohydrates: 1.4 g dietary fiber: 0 g**

Mushroom Quiche Canapés

Make crab canapés as above, substituting 2 tablespoons (30 mL) sautéed chopped mushrooms for the crabmeat.

  **calories: 15 total fat: 0.6 g saturated fat: 0.2 g cholesterol: 18 mg
  sodium: 19 mg carbohydrates: 1.4 g dietary fiber: 0 g**

Rolled Asparagus Canapés

Elegant! Use the softest high-fiber bread so it doesn't crack as you roll it.

10	thin slices of high-fiber bread	10
1 t	butter or margarine, softened	5 mL
1 t	fat-free mayonnaise	5 mL
10	canned asparagus spears, well drained	10

Cut the crusts off the bread slices. In a small bowl mix the butter and mayonnaise together. Spread each slice of bread thinly with the butter-mayonnaise mixture. Place an asparagus tip along the edge of a piece of bread and roll tightly. Repeat with each slice of bread. Arrange on a plate and cover with waxed paper until serving time.

Yield: 10 canapés

Each canapé contains:
calories: 87 total fat: 1.4 g saturated fat: 0.5 g cholesterol: 1 mg sodium: 142 mg carbohydrates: 15.5 g dietary fiber: 2.0 g

Salmon & Cream Cheese Roll-Ups

Serve on lettuce leaves for an elegant look.

| ¼ lb. | smoked salmon (lox) sliced | 100 g |
| 4 oz. | fat-free cream cheese | 100 g |

Lie the salmon slices flat. Spread each with cream cheese. Roll up, starting at the short end. Cut the rolls about ½ inch (1.3 cm) thick.

Yield: 18 roll-ups

Each roll-up contains:
calories: 13 total fat: 0.3 g saturated fat: 0.1 g cholesterol: 3 mg sodium: 79 mg carbohydrates: 0.4 g dietary fiber: 0 g

Quick Cucumber Sauce for Fish

A fresh, light flavor.

½ C	fat-free mayonnaise	125 mL
½ C	cucumber, finely chopped	125 mL
1 t	vinegar	5 mL
dash	Worcestershire sauce	dash
1 t	grated onion (optional)	5 mL

Combine all the ingredients and chill before serving.

Yield: 1 cup

Each tablespoon contains:
**calories: 7 total fat: 0 g saturated fat: 0 g cholesterol: 3 mg
sodium: 38 mg carbohydrates: 0.9 g dietary fiber: 0.2 g**

Low-Fat French Dressing

Nothing could be easier to throw together.

| ½ C | fat-free mayonnaise | 125 mL |
| 2 T | ketchup | 30 mL |

Place the mayonnaise and ketchup in a small bowl and mix together thoroughly.

Yield: ¾ cup

Each tablespoon contains:
**calories: 26 total fat: 1.9 g saturated fat: 0.3 g cholesterol: 2 mg
sodium: 79 mg carbohydrates: 2.3 g dietary fiber: 0 g**

Yogurt-Dill Dressing

Try this dressing on salads and fish.

1 C	nonfat yogurt	250 mL
¼ C	onion, very finely chopped	60 mL
¼ t	dried dill	2 mL
2 T	Parmesan cheese	30 mL

Combine the ingredients in a blender or food processor until smooth.

Yield: 1¼ C

Each tablespoon contains:
**calories: 11 total fat: 0.2 g saturated fat: 0.1 g cholesterol: 1 mg
sodium: 27 mg carbohydrates: 1.3 g dietary fiber: 0 g**

Low-Fat Russian Dressing

Serve over your favorite salad.

½ C	fat-free mayonnaise	125 mL
2 T	ketchup	30 mL
2 T	relish	30 mL

Place the ingredients in a small bowl. Combine thoroughly using a fork.

Yield: ¾ cup

Each tablespoon contains:
**calories: 12 total fat: 0 g saturated fat: 0 g cholesterol: 4 mg
sodium: 80 mg carbohydrates: 1.8 g dietary fiber: 0.3 g**

Low-Fat California Dip

My daughter Anna's favorite dip. It's not a party without it!

| 16 oz. | nonfat sour cream | 454 g |
| 1 envelope | dried onion-soup mix | 1 envelope |

Blend the sour cream and onion-soup mix together. Chill.

Yield: 2 cups

Each tablespoon contains:

calories: 13 **total fat:** 0.1 g **saturated fat:** 0 g **cholesterol:** 0 mg
sodium: 121 mg **carbohydrates:** 2 g **dietary fiber:** 0.1 g

Bread Bowl Spinach Dip

Low-fat version of the dip our friend Peg always serves at her holiday party.

10 oz. pkg.	frozen spinach, thawed and well drained	284 t
¼ C	onion, finely chopped(optional)	60 mL
¼ C	parsley, finely chopped	60 mL
1 C	fat-free sour cream	250 mL
1 C	fat-free cream cheese, whipped	250 mL
8 oz. can	water chestnuts, drained and chopped	227 g can
1	round loaf of bread, unsliced	1

Combine all the ingredients except the bread. Chill. Take a slice off the top of the bread and scoop out the center. Cut the removed bread into cubes. Fill the hole in the bread with the dip. Serve the bread cubes on the side.

Yield: 3½ cups of dip

Each tablespoon contains:

calories: 71 **total fat:** 0.7 g **saturated fat:** 0.1 g **cholesterol:** 2 mg
sodium: 156 mg **carbohydrates:** 12.5 g **dietary fiber:** 1.0 g

Salmon Dip

Serve with chunks of fresh bagel.

1 (15 oz.) can	salmon	1 (425 g) can
¼ C	onion, finely chopped (optional)	60 mL
1 t	Worcestershire sauce	5 mL
1 C	fat-free sour cream	250 mL

Place all the ingredients except the sour cream in a blender or food processor. On low speed, process to mix the ingredients. Transfer to a mixing bowl. Mix in the sour cream. Chill before serving.

Yield: 1½ cups

Each tablespoon contains:
**calories: 28 total fat: 0.6 g saturated fat: 0.1 g cholesterol: 9 mg
sodium: 29 mg carbohydrates: 1.1 g dietary fiber: 0 g**

Clam Dip

Serve with low-fat chips or vegetables for dipping.

1 C	fat-free sour cream	250 mL
½ C	fat-free cream cheese	125 mL
2 t	Worcestershire sauce	10 mL
8 oz. can	minced clams, drained	227 g

Blend together the sour cream, cream cheese, and Worcestershire sauce. Add the clams and stir until evenly distributed. Chill. Note: if dip is too thick, thin with a tablespoon (15 mL) of skim milk just before serving.

Yield: 1½ cups (24 servings)

Each serving contains:
**calories: 19 total fat: 0.1 g saturated fat: 0 g cholesterol: 4 mg
sodium: 50 mg carbohydrates: 18 g dietary fiber: 0 g**

Eggplant Dip

This is a delicious and unusual dip.

1	eggplant, washed and dried, skin and stem intact	1
¼ C	tahini (sesame seed paste)	60 mL
¼ C	lemon juice	60 mL
2 t	olive oil	10 mL
1 T	parsley, finely chopped	15 mL

Use a fork to pierce the eggplant several times. Place on a foil-lined baking sheet and bake in a preheated 350°F (180°C) oven for one hour. Set in sink under cool running water. Remove the skin and stem. Place in a colander to drain well. Transfer the eggplant to a mixing bowl. Use a fork to mash the eggplant. Add the rest of the ingredients and mix until blended.

Yield: 2 cups

Each tablespoon contains:
**calories: 19 total fat: 1.3 g saturated fat: 0.2 g cholesterol: 0 mg
sodium: 1 mg carbohydrates: 1.6 g dietary fiber: 0.5 g**

Stuffed Snow Peas

Beautiful!

30	fresh snow pea pods	30
¼ C	fat-free soft cream cheese	60 mL
⅛ t	dried dill weed	1 mL
1 T	fresh parsley, chopped fine	15 mL

Immerse the pea pods in rapidly boiling water for 10 seconds. Drain them in a colander, rinsing with cold water to cool them rapidly and stop them from cooking. Using a sharp knife, open the pods along the end. In a small mixing bowl combine the remaining ingredients. Insert ½ t (3 mL) of cream cheese mixture into each pod.

Yield: 20 pods

Each pod contains:
**calories: 65 total fat: 0.4 g saturated fat: 0.1 g cholesterol: 0 mg
sodium: 366 mg carbohydrates: 10.8 g dietary fiber: 4.2 g**

Pistachio-Stuffed Celery

A real treat! Your guests will love them.

½ C	fat-free cream cheese	125 mL
½ t	Worcestershire sauce	3 mL
½ t	lemon juice	3 mL
1 T	pistachio nuts, chopped fine	15 mL
24	celery pieces, each one inch (2.5 cm) long	24

Mix together the cream cheese, Worcestershire sauce, and lemon juice. Stir in the nuts. Spoon the cream cheese mixture into the hollows of the celery pieces.

Yield: 24 pieces

Each tablespoon contains:

**calories: 8 total fat: 0.2 g saturated fat: 0 g cholesterol: 1 mg
sodium: 32 mg carbohydrates: 0.8 g dietary fiber: 0.2 g**

Clam Sauce for Pasta

Use this instead of tomato-based sauce for pasta.

14 oz.	clams; reserving the juice	400 g
3	cloves of garlic, peeled and chopped (optional)	3
⅓ C	olive oil	80 mL
¼ C	parsley, chopped	60 mL

Drain the clams, reserving the juice. Chop the clams and set them aside. Sauté the garlic, if you are using it, in the olive oil. Add the clam juice to the oil and heat without boiling. Add the parsley and clams. Toss with cooked noodles or spaghetti. Serve hot with grated Parmesan or Romano cheese.

Yield: 4 servings

Each serving contains:
**calories: 246 total fat: 19.2 g saturated fat: 2.5 g cholesterol: 34 mg
sodium: 73 mg carbohydrates: 5.3 g dietary fiber: 0.4 g**

Chapter 8
DESSERTS

Cherry Torte

A cherry lover's favorite.

1	egg or equivalent egg substitute	1
1 C	sugar	250 mL
2 C	pitted sour cherries, drained	500 mL
1 C	flour	250 mL
¼ t	salt	2 mL
½ t	baking soda	3 mL
1 T	butter or margarine, melted	15 mL
1 t	almond extract	5 mL
½ C	walnuts, chopped (optional)	125 mL

Beat the egg, gradually adding the sugar until it dissolves. Carefully fold in the cherries. In another bowl, sift together the flour, salt, and baking soda. Fold the dry ingredients into the cherry-egg mixture. Gently mix in the butter and the almond extract. Pour into a 9 inch (22 cm) round pan coated with a nonstick cooking spray. Sprinkle the nuts over the top, if desired. Bake in a preheated 350°F (180°C) oven for 45 minutes.

Yield: 8 servings

Each serving contains:
**calories: 201 total fat: 2.6 g saturated fat: 1.2 g cholesterol: 30 mg
sodium: 173 mg carbohydrates: 42.6 g dietary fiber: 0.5 g**

Berry Torte

Very European!

16	graham crackers	16
½ C	sugar	125 mL
¼ C	butter or margarine, melted	60 mL
2	eggs or equivalent egg substitute	2
8 oz.	nonfat cream cheese, softened	200 g
½ C	sugar	125 mL
10 oz.	nonfat frozen raspberries, blueberries, or strawberries—reserving the juice when thawing	284 g
1 T	lemon juice	15 mL
½ C	sugar (optional)	125 mL
1 T	cornstarch	15 mL

Process the graham crackers in a blender or food processor until they are reduced to crumbs. Pour them into a bowl. Add the sugar and the melted butter. Toss and stir with a fork until combined. Press the mixture into a 9 inch (22 cm) square pan using your hands. Cover the bottom of the pan. Put the eggs and cream cheese into a blender or food processor. Blend until they are combined and smooth. Add the next ½ C (125 mL) sugar while blending. Spread the cream cheese mixture over the graham crackers. Bake in a preheated 350°F (180°C) oven for 25 minutes. Set on a wire rack to cool.

In a small saucepan, combine 1 C (250 mL) of the reserved berry juice, the lemon juice, and the cornstarch. Use a wire whisk to stir. Cook, stirring constantly, until mixture is thick and translucent. Spread over the cooled cheese mixture. Chill.

Yield: 9 servings

Each serving contains:
**calories: 241 total fat: 7.6 g saturated fat: 3.8 g cholesterol: 65 mg
sodium: 261 mg carbohydrates: 38.3 g dietary fiber: 2.5 g**

Wild Blueberry Torte

Originally intended for those tiny wild blueberries, this torte works just as well with the larger frozen ones.

½ C	flour	125 mL
1 t	baking powder	5 mL
½ C	sugar	125 mL
2	eggs or equivalent egg substitute	2
1 t	almond extract	5 mL
1 t	vanilla extract	5 mL
2 C	blueberries (frozen are fine)	500 mL

Sift together the flour and baking powder into a medium mixing bowl. Stir in the sugar. In another bowl, mix together the eggs and extracts. Add the blueberries to the flour mixture and mix gently. Gently fold in the wet mixture. Pour into an 8 inch (20 cm) square pan that has been coated with a nonstick cooking spray. Bake in a preheated 350°F (180°C) oven for 35-40 minutes.

Yield: 9 pieces

Each piece contains:
**calories: 104 total fat: 1.3 g saturated fat: 0.4 g cholesterol: 47 mg
sodium: 57 mg carbohydrates: 21.3 g dietary fiber: 0.9 g**

Apple Crisp

Good warm or cold anytime.

4 C	apples, sliced	1 L
1 T	lemon juice	15 mL
¼ C	flour	60 mL
¾ C	"old fashioned" oatmeal (not quick-cooking)	185 mL
2 T	brown sugar	30 mL
3 T	white sugar	45 mL
1 t	cinnamon	5 mL
6 T	butter or margarine	90 mL
dash	cloves	dash

Arrange the apple slices in a baking pan and sprinkle with the lemon juice. In a bowl combine the remaining ingredients to make a crumbly mixture. Spoon the mixture over the apples. Bake in a 375°F (190°C) oven for 30 minutes.

Yield: 6 servings

Each serving contains:
**calories: 222 total fat: 11.8 g saturated fat: 7.1 g cholesterol: 31 mg
sodium: 171 mg carbohydrates: 29.3 g dietary fiber: 2.4 g**

Fruit Slump

An old pioneer recipe. There is nothing tricky about making it.

4 C	apple slices, cored and peeled	1 L
½ C	sugar	125 mL
½ t	ginger or cinnamon (optional)	3 mL
1 C	flour	250 mL
1½ t	baking powder	3 mL
¼ C	sugar	60 mL
¾ C	skim milk	185 mL
2 T	butter or margarine, melted	30 mL
2 T	olive oil	30 mL

Arrange the apple slices in an 8 inch (20 cm) baking pan. Sprinkle the ½ C (125 mL) sugar and the spices, if desired, over the apples and toss to coat. In a mixing bowl, combine the flour, baking powder, and sugar. Stir in the rest of the ingredients to make a batter. Pour the batter over the fruit and bake in a preheated 375°F (190°C) oven for 45 minutes. Serve hot or warm.

Yield: 4 servings

Each serving contains:
**calories: 451 total fat: 13.2 g saturated fat: 4.6 g cholesterol: 16 mg
sodium: 219 mg carbohydrates: 81.0 g dietary fiber: 3.0 g**

Fruit Salad Cake

This low-fat cake is moist and delicious.

1 C	flour	250 mL
1 t	baking soda	5 mL
½ t	salt	3 mL
1 C	sugar	250 mL
½ C	walnuts (optional)	125 mL
1	egg or equivalent egg substitute, lightly beaten	1
1 t	almond extract	5 mL
1 t	vanilla extract	5 mL
16 oz. can	"lite" fruit cocktail, packed in juice	454 g
½ C	brown sugar	125 mL

In a large mixing bowl, mix together the flour, baking soda, salt, sugar, and nuts, if desired. In another bowl, mix together the egg, extracts, and can of fruit cocktail (including the juice) carefully until just blended. Pour the fruit cocktail mixture over the dry ingredients and stir to combine just until moist. Pour into an 8 inch (20 cm) square pan that has been coated with a nonstick cooking spray. Sprinkle the top with the brown sugar. Bake in a preheated 350°F (180°C) oven for 45 minutes.

Yield: 12 squares

Each square contains:
**calories: 149 total fat: 0.5 g saturated fat: 0.2 g cholesterol: 18 mg
sodium: 203 mg carbohydrates: 35.1 g dietary fiber: 0.4 g**

Strawberry Layer Cake

This unusual cake is made in a frying pan!

3	eggs or equivalent egg substitute	3
½ C	sugar	125 mL
1 C	flour	250 mL
2 t	baking powder	10 mL
8 T	butter or margarine, melted	120 mL
1 C	applesauce	250 mL
10 oz.	frozen strawberries, defrosted and drained	284 g

Lightly oil a 6 to 8 inch (15-20 cm) skillet or griddle and heat it over a low flame on the top of the stove. Beat the eggs and sugar in a mixing bowl on high speed until they are thick. Sift together the flour and baking powder. Add to the egg and sugar, mixing gently by hand. Add the butter and mix gently. Pour about ½ cup (125 mL) of batter into the heated skillet; the batter should cover the bottom of the pan and be about the thickness of a pancake. Bake in the oven five minutes until the cake is lightly browned. Use a spatula to remove the layer to a serving plate. Pour another ½ cup (125 mL) of batter into the skillet and repeat, making three layers in all. Blend the strawberries and applesauce together. Spread a layer of fruit between each of the three layers and on top. Serve within 6 hours for best results.

Yield: 8 servings

Each serving contains:
**calories: 269 total fat: 13.6 g saturated fat: 7.7 g cholesterol: 110 mg
sodium: 232 mg carbohydrates: 33.8 g dietary fiber: 1.2 g**

Pineapple Upside-Down Cake

My favorite birthday cake.

⅓ C	brown sugar	80 mL
1 t	cinnamon	5 mL
5 slices	pineapple slices	5 slices
(7 oz.)		(200 g)
1 C	flour	250 mL
1 T	baking powder	15 mL
½ C	sugar	125 mL
1	egg or equivalent egg substitute	1
¼ C	skim milk	60 mL
3 T	butter or margarine	45 mL

Oil an 8 inch (20 cm) round cake pan or coat it with a nonstick spray. Combine the brown sugar and cinnamon in a small bowl and sprinkle the mixture evenly on the bottom of the pan. Arrange the pineapple slices on top of the sugar. Sift together the flour and baking powder in a large mixing bowl. Add the sugar, egg, milk, and melted margarine. Beat until well mixed. Pour the batter on top of the pineapple slices. Bake in a 350°F (180°C) oven about 30 minutes, or until a cake tester or toothpick inserted into the center comes out clean. Cool for about 10 to 15 minutes. Loosen the sides and put a plate upside down over the cake. Invert and remove pan.

Yield: 8 servings

Each serving contains:
**calories: 136 total fat: 2.6 g saturated fat: 1.5 g cholesterol: 19 mg
sodium: 98 mg carbohydrates: 28.0 g dietary fiber: 0.6 g**

Low-Cal Vanilla Cake

This mock pound cake is delicious with fresh fruit.

2	eggs or equivalent egg substitute	2
⅔ C	sugar	160 mL
⅔ C	flour	160 mL
1 t	baking powder	5 mL
3 T	hot water	45 mL
1 t	vanilla extract	5 mL
1 T	butter or margarine, melted	15 mL
1 t	canola or safflower oil	5 mL
1 t	bread crumbs	5 mL

Using an electric mixer, beat the eggs in a mixing bowl. Gradually add the sugar and continue beating until the mixture is light. Sift together the flour and baking powder. In a small bowl, mix the hot water and vanilla together. To the egg mixture in the mixing bowl add half the flour, then the hot water, then the rest of the flour, stirring after each addition. Fold in the butter and oil. Coat a loaf pan with nonstick cooking spray and dust it with bread crumbs. Turn the batter into the prepared loaf pan. Bake in a preheated 350°F (180°C) oven for 40 minutes. The top of the cake will spring back when pressed lightly. Cool on a wire rack.

Yield: 12 slices

Each slice contains:
**calories: 85 total fat: 1.3 g saturated fat: 0.3 g cholesterol: 35 mg
sodium: 42 mg carbohydrates: 16.8 g dietary fiber: 0 g**

Angel Food Cake

Don't use a knife to cut angel food cake. Pull apart the slices with opposing forks.

1 C	sifted cake flour	250 mL
1 C	sugar	250 mL
¼ t	salt	2 mL
1⅓ C	egg whites (usually one dozen)	330 mL
1 t	cream of tartar	5 mL
1 t	vanilla extract	5 mL
1 t	almond extract	5 mL

Sift the cake flour with one-quarter cup of the sugar and the salt. Sift the mixture about four or five times. Beat the egg whites, using an electric mixer. Add the cream of tartar when the egg whites are foamy, but beat until the egg whites form stiff, but not dry, peaks. Beat in the vanilla, almond extract, and the rest of the sugar a tablespoon (15 mL) at a time. Carefully fold in the flour mixture ¼ C (60 mL) at a time. Pour into an ungreased angel cake pan (9 inch—22 cm—tube pan). Bake in a preheated 325°F (160°C) oven. Check after 40 minutes to see if top is browned. Bake up to 60 minutes until top is lightly browned. Remove from the oven and invert on a wire rack for 60 minutes to cool. Use a spatula to remove the cake from the pan if necessary.

Yield: 16 slices

Each slice contains:
**calories: 84 total fat: 0.1 g saturated fat: 0 g cholesterol: 0 mg
sodium: 67 mg carbohydrates: 18 g dietary fiber: 0.1 g**

Apple Cake

Good for dessert or for snacking.

⅔ C	canola oil	170 mL
½ C	sugar	125 mL
1	egg or equivalent egg substitute, lightly beaten	1
1 t	vanilla extract	5 mL
1 t	almond extract	5 mL
½ t	baking soda	3 mL
1 t	baking powder	5 mL
1½ C	flour	375 mL
½ C	raisins	125 mL
1½ C	apples, diced	375 mL
2 T	chopped nuts (optional)	30 mL

In a large mixing bowl, combine the oil, sugar, egg, and vanilla and almond extracts. In a second bowl, mix the baking soda and baking powder with the flour. Add this dry mixture to the wet mixture and stir to moisten. Mix in the raisins and apples. Sprinkle the nuts over the top, if desired. Turn the mixture into a 9 inch (22 cm) square pan that has been coated with a nonstick cooking spray. Bake in a pre-heated 350°F (180°C) oven for 30 minutes. Cut into 16 pieces.

Yield: 16 servings

Each serving contains:

**calories: 172 total fat: 9.6 g saturated fat: 0.8 g cholesterol: 13 mg
sodium: 16 mg carbohydrates: 20.5 g dietary fiber: 0.5 g**

"Creamy" Rice Pudding

Serve this traditional favorite warm or cold.

2 C	1% (low-fat) milk	500 mL
dash	salt	salt
½ C	white rice, rinsed and drained	125 mL
1	egg	1
½ C	evaporated milk	125 mL
1 t	vanilla extract	5 mL
¼ C	sugar	60 mL
½ C	raisins, soaked in hot water	125 mL
	for 15 minutes and drained	

In a medium saucepan over low heat slowly warm the milk. Add the salt and rice and stir. Bring to a slow boil, then reduce the heat to simmer. Cook until the rice is soft (about 15 minutes) stirring occasionally. While the rice is cooking, blend the eggs and ¼ C (60 mL) of the evaporated milk, vanilla, and sugar together in a mixing bowl. Set aside. When the rice begins to get soft, add the remainder of the evaporated milk and the raisins. Stir. Spoon a few spoonfuls of rice mixture into the egg mixture. Stir and pour the egg mixture into the saucepan, stir and return to the heat. Cook, stirring until the pudding becomes bubbly and thick. Pour into four serving dishes. Refrigerate the pudding if it is not being served right away.

Yield: 4 servings

Each serving contains:
**calories: 300 total fat: 5.2 g saturated fat: 2.7 g cholesterol: 67 mg
sodium: 114 mg carbohydrates: 54.6 g dietary fiber: 1.0 g**

Southern Classic Banana Pudding

Equally good warm or chilled!

3	eggs, separated	3
1	egg or equivalent egg substitute, beaten	3
½ C	sugar	125 mL
3 T	flour	45 mL
2 C	nonfat milk	500 mL
½ t	vanilla	3 mL
3 oz.	vanilla wafers	85 g
6	medium ripe bananas, peeled and sliced	6
¼ C	sugar	60 mL

In the top of a double boiler, combine the egg yolks and the beaten egg with the sugar and flour. Stir in the milk. Cook over boiling water, stirring constantly until it is thickened. It is ready when spoon marks in the custard are visible while you stir. Stir in the vanilla and remove from heat. Spread a small amount of the custard on the bottom of a 1½ quart (1.5 L) casserole dish. Layer the wafers, which should lie flat, with the layer of sliced bananas. Pour about one-third of the custard over the bananas. Continuing layering wafers, bananas, and custard to make three layers of each. End with a custard layer. Beat the three egg whites until stiff. Gradually add the remaining the ¼ C (60 mL) sugar. Beat until the mixture forms stiff peaks. Spoon the meringue on top of pudding. Cover the entire surface. Bake in a preheated 425°F (220°C) oven about 5 minutes or so, until the meringue is delicately brown.

Yield: 8 servings

Each serving contains:
**calories: 278 total fat: 5.4 g saturated fat: 1.6 g cholesterol: 107 mg
sodium: 101 mg carbohydrates: 52.9 g dietary fiber: 2.1 g**

Prune-Apricot Pudding

Moist enough to be a pudding but bakes like a cake.

1 C	sifted flour	250 mL
1 t	baking soda	5 mL
1 C	raisins (optional)	250 mL
1 C	walnuts, chopped (optional)	250 mL
1 C	sugar	250 mL
½ C	cooked apricots, mashed	125 mL
½ C	cooked prunes, mashed	125 mL
1 T	butter, melted	15 mL
1 t	vanilla	5 mL
¾ C	nonfat milk	185 mL

Sift the flour and baking soda together. Add the raisins and walnuts, if desired. In another bowl, combine the sugar, apricots, and prunes with the butter, vanilla, and milk. Add the flour mixture and mix thoroughly. Pour the pudding into an 8 inch (20 cm) square pan that has been coated with a nonstick cooking spray. Bake in a preheated 325°F (160°C) oven for 1 hour.

Yield: 9 servings

Each serving contains:
calories: 180 total fat: 1.5 g saturated fat: 0.8 g cholesterol: 4 mg sodium: 164 mg carbohydrates: 40 g dietary fiber: 0.9 g

Colonial Indian Pudding

Serve warm or cold.

1 C	molasses	250 mL
2 T	butter or margarine, melted	30 mL
½ t	salt	3 mL
10 T	cornmeal	150 mL
2	eggs or equivalent egg substitute, beaten	2
4 C	nonfat milk	1 L

In a mixing bowl, stir together the molasses, melted butter, and salt. Add the cornmeal and mix. Set aside. In a saucepan, bring the milk just to the boiling point. Stir gradually into the molasses mixture. Pour into a 1½ quart (1.5 L) baking dish. Bake in a 325°F (160°C) oven for 90 minutes or until the pudding is set.

Yield: 8 servings

Each serving contains:
**calories: 235 total fat: 4.5 g saturated fat: 2.3 g cholesterol: 63 mg
sodium: 256 mg carbohydrates: 42.7 g dietary fiber: 0.8 g**

Scandinavian Pudding

No, pineapples are not native to Scandinavia, but this dessert is a favorite.

6 oz.	frozen pineapple juice concentrate	180 g
2½ C	water	625 mL
4 T	farina	60 mL
8 oz.	crushed pineapple, packed in its juice, drained	200 g

Mix the pineapple concentrate and water in a small saucepan. Bring to a rapid boil. Stir the mixture while gradually adding the farina.

Cook gently for five minutes or so; remove from heat. Beat by hand or with an electric mixer until the mixture is smooth. Fold in the pineapple. Pour into individual serving dishes, chill.

Yield: 6 servings

Each serving contains:
**calories: 100 total fat: 0.1 g saturated fat: 0 g cholesterol: 0 mg
sodium: 1 mg carbohydrates: 24.2 g dietary fiber: 0.5 g**

Vanilla Pudding

If you're used to pudding mixes, you will be pleasantly surprised at how easy this is.

2 C	skim milk	500 mL
2 T	butter or margarine	30 mL
3 T	cornstarch	45 mL
½ C	sugar	125 mL
1	egg or equivalent egg substitute	1
1 T	vanilla extract	15 mL

Heat the milk and the margarine in the top of a double boiler over simmering water. In a bowl, mix together the cornstarch and sugar. Add the eggs or substitute and blend well. Add the vanilla and blend. Pour the cornstarch mixture into the warm milk. Mix with a wire whisk over simmering water until the mixture is thick. A good way to know if it's done is to look for wire whisk patterns; if they stay in the pudding it's done. Cool pudding before serving.

Yield: 4 servings

Each serving contains:
**calories: 235 total fat: 7.2 g saturated fat: 4.1 g cholesterol: 71 mg
sodium: 137 mg carbohydrates: 36.9 g dietary fiber: 0.1 g**

"Leftover Muffin" Pudding

Make this with homemade or store-bought muffins. Staleness doesn't matter.

4	fat-free muffins	4
3	apples, peeled and sliced	3
3	ripe bananas	3
¾ C	nonfat milk	185 mL
1 t	vanilla extract	5 mL
1 t	almond extract	5 mL
2	egg whites	2
¼ C	sugar	60 mL

Crumble the muffins into a large mixing bowl. Gently stir in the apples, bananas, milk, and extracts and let stand. In another bowl, beat the egg whites until stiff, add the sugar gradually, and keep beating until stiff and glossy. Fold into the muffin mixture and spoon into a 1 quart (1 L) baking pan coated with a nonstick cooking spray. Bake in a preheated 350°F (180°C) oven for 30 minutes. The top will be lightly browned.

Yield: 6 servings

Each serving contains:
**calories: 363 total fat: 0.6 g saturated fat: 0.2 g cholesterol: 1 mg
sodium: 395 mg carbohydrates: 87.2 g dietary fiber: 4.6 g**

Grape Nuts Pudding

Making a comeback in restaurants.

2	eggs or equivalent egg substitute	2
1 C	sugar	250 mL
1 C	Grape Nuts cereal	250 mL
4 C	nonfat milk	1 L

| 1 t | vanilla | 5 mL |
| 1 T | butter or margarine | 15 mL |

Beat eggs and gradually add the sugar, beating until it is dissolved. Mix in the Grape Nuts, milk, and vanilla. Pour into a 1½ quart (1.5 L) baking dish that has been coated with a nonstick cooking spray. Dot the top with the butter. Bake in a preheated 350°F (180°C) oven for 1 hour. Serve warm or cold.

Yield: 8 servings

Each serving contains:
calories: 165 total fat: 1.5 g saturated fat: 0.4 g cholesterol: 53 mg sodium: 103 mg carbohydrates: 36.9 g dietary fiber: 1.3 g

Apple Tapioca

If you like tapioca, you'll love this recipe.

⅓ C	quick-cooking tapioca	80 mL
2⅔ C	boiling water	670 mL
4	apples, peeled, cored, and quartered	4
⅔ C	sugar	170 mL
1 T	butter or margarine	15 mL

Stir the tapioca into the boiling water and cook for 10 minutes. The mixture will be clear. Arrange the apples in a small casserole dish. Sprinkle the sugar over the apples. Dot with butter. Pour the cooked tapioca over the apples. Bake in a preheated 350°F (180°C) oven for 20 minutes or until apples are soft.

Yield: 4 servings

Each serving contains:
calories: 278 total fat: 3.3 g saturated fat: 1.9 g cholesterol: 8 mg sodium: 34 mg carbohydrates: 65.6 g dietary fiber: 3.8 g

Bananas Foster

A spectacular yet easy dessert topping that is traditionally served over vanilla ice cream. This recipe is so delicious, you may prefer it without the ice cream. It can also be served over lemon sherbet or waffles.

4	ripe bananas	4
2 t	lemon juice	10 mL
4 T	butter or margarine	60 mL
2 T	brown sugar	30 mL
dash	cinnamon	dash
1 T	white sugar	15 mL
¼ C	light rum	60 mL

Peel the bananas; then cut them lengthwise and across into four pieces. Sprinkle with lemon juice. In a chafing dish melt the margarine over low heat. Stir in the brown sugar and cinnamon. Add the bananas and cook for approximately two minutes, stirring without crushing the bananas. Sprinkle with sugar and add the rum. Use a long wooden match and ignite the rum. Serve as soon as it burns itself out.

Yield: 4 servings

Each serving contains:
**calories: 267 total fat: 11.9 g saturated fat: 7.3 g cholesterol: 31 mg
sodium: 119 mg carbohydrates: 34.5 g dietary fiber: 2.8 g**

Baked Banana in Skins

You can also grill bananas on your outdoor grill.

4	bananas	4
sprinkle	confectioners' sugar	sprinkle

Place bananas in their skins on a foil-lined baking pan (The foil is for easy clean-up). Bake in a preheated 375°F (190°C) oven for 20 minutes. Peel and sprinkle with confectioners' sugar.

Yield: 4 servings

Each serving contains:
**calories: 105 total fat: 0.6 g saturated fat: 0.2 g cholesterol: 0 mg
sodium: 1 mg carbohydrates: 26.7 g dietary fiber: 2.7 g**

Baked Banana

Why not?

1	medium banana	1
1 t	lemon juice	5 mL
1 T	honey	15 mL

Cut banana in half the long way. Put the halves cut side up in a baking dish. Mix the lemon juice and honey together and brush over the banana halves. Bake uncovered in a preheated 400°F (200°C) oven for 10 minutes until the banana is golden.

Yield: 2 servings

Each serving contains:
**calories: 85 total fat: 0.3 g saturated fat: 0.1 g cholesterol: 0 mg
sodium: 1 mg carbohydrates: 22.3 g dietary fiber: 1.4 g**

Mandarin Orange Gelatin-Sherbet

Turns orange sherbet into a special dessert.

11 oz.	canned mandarin oranges	310 g
1 env. (1 T)	plain gelatin	1 env. (15 mL)
2 T	sugar	30 mL
1 C	orange sherbet	250 mL

Drain the liquid from a can of oranges and reserve the oranges. Combine the liquid with enough water to make 1 cup (250 mL). Bring to a boil. Dissolve the gelatin and sugar in the liquid. Stir in the sherbet and the oranges and cook over low heat until dissolved. If you like, use two drops each of red and yellow food coloring. Spray a mold with nonstick cooking spray; pour gelatin into the mold; chill. To unmold, briefly place in warm water, place an upside-down serving plate over the mold, and turn both over simultaneously. Lift off the mold.

Yield: 4 servings

Each serving contains:
   **calories: 131   total fat: 1.0 g   saturated fat: 0.6 g   cholesterol: 4 mg
sodium: 31 mg   carbohydrates: 30 g   dietary fiber: 0.5 g**

Cool Strawberry Fluff

A light and lovely way to top off a meal.

10 oz.	strawberries, sliced (fresh or frozen)	284 g
2 env. (2 T)	unflavored gelatin	30 mL
1 C	coarsely crushed ice	250 mL

Drop ½ cup (125 mL) of the strawberries into a blender container and blend for about five seconds. Transfer the strawberries to a small saucepan, warm over low heat until they begin to boil, then pour into the blender. Sprinkle the gelatin over the hot strawberries, cover, and blend for 30 seconds. Add the crushed ice and blend on a low speed for about 20 seconds. Switch to a high speed and blend for about 30 seconds more. Place the remaining strawberries in a bowl and add the blended mixture. Pour into individual dishes or a serving bowl. Chill.

Yield: 4 servings

Each serving contains:
calories: 42 total fat: 0.4 g saturated fat: 0 g cholesterol: 0 mg
sodium: 13 mg carbohydrates: 8.3 g dietary fiber: 1.6 g

Orange Cream

A luscious way to serve canned fruit.

2 pkg.	sugar-free orange gelatin mix (4-serving size)	2 pkg.
2 C	canned pears, drained and diced	500 mL
1	egg yolk	1
1 T	sugar	15 mL
1 t	cornstarch	5 mL
¾ C	skim milk	185 mL
1 t	vanilla extract	5 mL

Prepare the gelatin according to the package directions. Coat six individual dessert cups with nonstick cooking spray. Distribute the fruit among the dessert cups and pour the gelatin over the fruit. Chill until firm. In a saucepan, mix the egg yolk, sugar, and cornstarch. Gradually add the milk, stirring constantly, and cook over low heat until the sauce thickens. Add the vanilla, stir, and cool. Unmold the gelatin onto dessert dishes. Place the sauce in a pitcher and pour it over each orange-gelatin portion.

Yield: 6 servings

Each serving contains:
calories: 161 total fat: 1.2 g saturated fat: 0.3 g cholesterol: 36 mg
sodium: 82 mg carbohydrates: 12.5 g dietary fiber: 1.3 g

Low-Calorie Tortoni

A low-fat, low-calorie version of the traditional Italian dish.

½ C	evaporated skim milk	125 mL
2 T	ground almonds (or other nuts)	30 mL
1	egg white, from an uncracked, clean egg	1
¼ C	light brown sugar, packed	60 mL
½ t	rum extract	3 mL
2 T	coconut flakes	30 mL
8	halves of maraschino cherries	8

Put the evaporated skim milk into a metal mixing bowl. Place in the freezer for one hour. Ice crystals should form, but the milk should not be frozen. Toast the almonds by sprinkling them onto a dry, heated frying pan and stirring until they are aromatic and nicely browned. Set aside. In a mixing bowl, beat the egg white until stiff. Sprinkle on the brown sugar and beat again until the two are completely blended. With an electric mixer on high speed, beat the cold milk until stiff. Beat in the rum extract. Fold in one tablespoon (15 mL) of the coconut and one tablespoon (15 mL) of the almonds. Fold this milk mixture into the egg white mixture until well blended. Spoon into the paper cups. Sprinkle each tortoni with the reserved almonds and coconut flakes. Top each one with a cherry half.

Yield: 8 servings

Each serving contains:
**calories: 196 total fat: 1.8 g saturated fat: 0.5 g cholesterol: 1 mg
sodium: 90 mg carbohydrates: 44.3 g dietary fiber: 1.4 g**

End of Summer Dessert

Luscious!

3 C	water	375 mL
½ C	sugar	125 mL
1	cinnamon stick	1
1	large apple, peeled, cored, and sliced	1
2	firm pears, peeled, pitted, and sliced	2
3	ripe peaches (dipped in boiling water to loosen skins, peeled, pitted, and sliced)	3

Bring the water, sugar, and cinnamon to a boil in a medium saucepan (not aluminum—it will stain). After five minutes, lower the heat to simmer and drop the apple slices into the water mixture. After 10 minutes drop in the pear slices. Simmer five minutes more before adding peach slices. Add the peaches and simmer for two more minutes. Cool and then refrigerate. Before serving, remove the cinnamon stick.

Yield: 4 servings

Each serving contains:
  **calories: 203 total fat: 0.6 g saturated fat: 0.1 g cholesterol: 0 mg
  sodium: 1 mg carbohydrates: 52.8 g dietary fiber: 6.1 g**

Pecan Meringues

Melts-in-your-mouth goodness.

1	egg white	1
1 C	light brown sugar, sifted	250 mL
1½ C	pecan halves	375 mL

Beat the egg white until it forms soft peaks. Continue beating, adding brown sugar gradually until the mixture is stiff. Fold in the pecan halves. Drop the batter by tablespoonfuls (15 mL) onto heavily greased baking sheets, spacing cookies an inch apart. Bake in a preheated 250°F (120°C) oven for 30 minutes until the cookies are pale brown. Remove the cookies onto cooling racks.

Yield: 24 cookies

Each cookie contains:
 **calories: 71 total fat: 4.8 g saturated fat: 0.4 g cholesterol: 9 mg
 sodium: 5 mg carbohydrates: 7.1 g dietary fiber: 0.5 g**

Meringue Miniatures

On damp days meringue can get chewy. These are still delicious.

2	egg whites	2
1 t	white vinegar	5 mL
½ t	almond extract	3 mL
½ t	vanilla extract	3 mL
½ C	sugar	125 mL

In a medium mixing bowl at high speed, beat the egg whites and vinegar until foamy and double in volume. Beat in the almond and vanilla extracts. Continue beating at high speed and gradually add the sugar until the meringue stands up in firm peaks. Line cookie sheets with parchment cooking paper or cut up brown-paper grocery bags. Drop the batter by teaspoonfuls onto the paper-lined cookie sheets, leaving an inch between cookies. Bake in a preheated 250°F (120°C) oven for 25 minutes. Lift the paper with the cookies on it onto a wire rack. After they have cooled completely, remove the cookies from the paper. It's important to store these cookies in an airtight container so they'll stay crisp.

Yield: 60 cookies

Each cookie contains:
 calories: 7 total fat: 0 g saturated fat: 0 g cholesterol: 0 mg
  sodium: 2 mg carbohydrates: 1.7 g dietary fiber: 0 g

Chocolate Chip Cookies

If the small amount of chocolate bothers you, try substituting carob chips.

1 C	flour	250 mL
2 t	baking powder	10 mL
8 T	butter or margarine	120 mL
½ t	vanilla extract	3 mL
¼ C	brown sugar	60 mL
½ C	sugar	125 mL
1	egg or equivalent egg substitute	1
1 C	chocolate chips	250 mL
½ C	walnuts, chopped (optional)	125 mL

Sift the flour and baking powder twice. Beat the margarine, vanilla, and sugars until fluffy and smooth. Beat in the egg. Add the flour mixture. Stir in the chips and nuts, if desired. Drop by teaspoonfuls onto a cookie sheet. Bake in a 375°F (190°C) oven about 10 minutes.

Yield: 50 cookies

Each cookie contains:
 calories: 61 total fat: 3.7 g saturated fat: 1.8 g cholesterol: 9 mg
  sodium: 35 mg carbohydrates: 7.0 g dietary fiber: 0.3 g

Pumpkin Cookies

Soft, moist cookies that pack well and stay fresh longer than other types of cookie.

1 C	butter or margarine, more for cookie sheets	250 mL
1 C	sugar	250 mL
1 C	canned pumpkin (not pumpkin pie filling)	250 mL
1	egg or equivalent egg substitute	1
1 t	vanilla extract	5 mL
2 C	flour	500 mL
2 T	baking powder	30 mL
1 t	cinnamon	5 mL
½ C	raisins	125 mL
½ C	unsalted walnuts, chopped	125 mL

Prepare your cookie sheets by coating them with nonstick spray or by rubbing them lightly with butter or margarine. Beat the butter until soft, gradually adding the sugar and beating until smooth. Add the pumpkin, egg, and vanilla. Mix well. In a bowl sift the flour, baking powder, and cinnamon together. Add the dry mixture to the pumpkin mixture; beat until smooth and rather fluffy. Stir in the raisins and chopped walnuts. Drop the batter by teaspoonfuls on cookie sheets. Bake in a 375°F (190°C) oven for 10 to 15 minutes.

Yield: 100 cookies

Each cookie contains:
> **calories: 40 total fat: 2.2 g saturated fat: 1.2 g cholesterol: 7 mg
> sodium: 41 mg carbohydrates: 4.7 g dietary fiber: 0.1 g**

Brownies

A cakelike brownie that keeps very well.

10 T	butter or margarine	150 mL
6 T	cocoa	90 mL
2	eggs or equivalent egg substitute	2
½ C	applesauce	125 mL
½C	sugar	125 mL
¼ C	brown sugar	60 mL
1 t	vanilla extract	5 mL
1 C	flour	250 mL
1½ t	baking powder	8 mL
½ C	walnuts, chopped	125 mL

Melt the butter, stir in the cocoa, and set aside. In a large bowl beat the eggs with a fork or a wire whisk. Add the applesauce, sugars, and vanilla and mix well. Mix the flour and baking powder and add to batter; stir well to blend. Add the cocoa mixture and the walnuts. Mix until well blended. Coat a 9 inch (22 cm) square pan with a nonstick spray. Bake in a 350°F (180°C) oven for 30 minutes or so, until a toothpick comes out clean. Cool and cut into 16 squares.

Yield: 16 servings

Each serving contains:
calories: 168 total fat: 10.3 g saturated fat: 4.9 g cholesterol: 46 mg sodium: 116 mg carbohydrates: 17.8 g dietary fiber: 1.0 g

Rice and Oatmeal Cookies

There is an extra crunchiness in these cookies.

1 C	butter or margarine	250 mL
½ C	white sugar	125 mL
½ C	brown sugar (packed)	125 mL
2	eggs or equivalent egg substitute, lightly beaten	2
1 t	vanilla extract	5 mL
2 C	flour	500 mL
1 t	baking soda	5 mL
½ t	baking powder	3 mL
2 C	oats, uncooked(not instant)	500 mL
2 C	rice cereal (such as Rice Krispies)	500 mL
1 C	coconut flakes	250 mL

Beat the butter in a medium mixing bowl until soft. Gradually add the sugars and continue beating until the mixture is fluffy and well blended. Add the eggs and vanilla. Mix well. In another bowl, mix together the flour, baking soda and baking powder. Combine the flour mixture with the butter mixture and blend well. Using a spoon, stir in the oats, rice cereal, and coconut. Use your hands to shape the batter into 1 inch (2.5 cm) balls. Coat a cookie sheet with nonstick cooking spray. Place the balls on the cookie sheet, leaving 2 inches (5 cm) between each. Flatten each slightly with a fork. Bake in a pre-heated 350°F (180°C) oven for 12 minutes. Carefully remove the cookies to a wire rack to cool.

Yield: 80 cookies

Each cookie contains:
**calories: 53 total fat: 2.8 g saturated fat: 0.7 g cholesterol: 5 mg
sodium: 68 mg carbohydrates: 6.5 g dietary fiber: 0.1 g**

Oatmeal Cookies

A traditional favorite.

¾ C	butter or margarine	185 mL
¾ C	brown sugar	185 mL
½ C	sugar	125 mL
1	egg or equivalent egg substitute	1
¼ C	water	60 mL
1 t	vanilla extract	5 mL
1 C	flour, sifted before being measured	250 mL
2 t	baking powder	10 mL
3 C	oats, uncooked (not instant or quick oats)	750 mL

Prepare cookie sheets by coating them with a nonstick spray. Combine the butter, sugars, egg, water, and vanilla in a mixing bowl. Beat until creamy. Sift together the flour and baking powder and add them to the mixing bowl; mix well. Add the oats and mix again. Drop by teaspoonfuls on cookie sheets; leaving about an inch or two (2.5–5 cm) room between each for the cookies to spread. Bake in a 350°F (180°C) oven 12 to 15 minutes. Cool for a minute before lifting them with a spatula and placing them on a cooling rack.

Yield: 80 cookies

Each cookie contains:
**calories: 38 total fat: 1.8 g saturated fat: 1.1 g cholesterol: 7 mg
sodium: 44 mg carbohydrates: 5.1 g dietary fiber: 0.1 g**

Raspberry Cream Puffs

You won't believe how easy cream puffs are to make.

2 T	butter or margarine, cut into pieces	30 mL
¼ C	water, boiling	60 mL
¼ C	flour	60 mL
1	egg or equivalent egg substitute	1
2 C	raspberries (drained frozen are fine)	500 mL
1 T	sugar	15 mL
¾ C	low-fat whipped topping	185 mL

Over medium heat in a small saucepan, mix the butter and boiling water. When it boils, add the flour and stir until the mixture forms a ball. Put the ball into a mixing bowl and add the egg. Beat until the mixture becomes satiny. Using a teaspoon, drop 18 blobs onto a cookie sheet that has been prepared with nonstick cooking spray. Bake in a preheated 375°F (190°C) oven for 20 minutes. Set on wire racks to cool. Mix the raspberries and sugar together. When you are ready to serve dessert, use a fork to split the puffs horizontally. Scoop raspberries between the puff halves, put the top back on and garnish with whipped topping.

Yield: 18 puffs

Each puff contains:
**calories: 37 total fat: 2.0 g saturated fat: 1.2 g cholesterol: 15 mg
sodium: 16 mg carbohydrates: 3.6 g dietary fiber: 0.9 g**

Thin Almond Wafers

Serve these with fat-free ice cream or even Jell-O!

2	egg whites	2
½ C	sugar	125 mL
⅓ C	flour	80 mL
¼ C	canola oil	60 mL
1 T	vanilla extract	15 mL
1 t	butter-flavored extract	5 mL
1 t	almond-flavored extract	5 mL

In a medium mixing bowl, mix together all the ingredients until just blended. Cover the bowl with plastic wrap and refrigerate for one hour. Line two cookie sheets with parchment baking paper (or, if you don't have baking paper, coat the sheets generously with nonstick cooking spray). Drop level teaspoonfuls of batter onto the cookie sheets. Space them evenly, about 12 per sheet. Gently smooth the batter into thin circles, using a butter knife or rubber spatula. Bake in a preheated 325°F (160°C) oven for 10 to 12 minutes. Cool on a wire rack. When cooled, store in airtight containers.

Yield: 24 cookies

Each cookie contains:
**calories: 44 total fat: 2.3 g saturated fat: 0.2 g cholesterol: 0 mg
sodium: 5 mg carbohydrates: 5.6 g dietary fiber: 0 g**

Apple Soufflés

Don't let the name scare you—this recipe is really easy.

1½ C	applesauce	375 mL
1 t	vanilla extract	5 mL
4	egg whites	4
½ C	sugar	125 mL
1T	sugar	15 mL

Mix together the applesauce and the vanilla extract. In a mixing bowl, beat the egg whites until foamy using an electric mixer. Gradually add the ½ C (125 mL) sugar beating continuously until the mixture is white, thick, and glossy. Fold into the applesauce mixture. Prepare six individual custard cups or glass baking dishes by coating them with a nonstick cooking spray. Spoon the egg white-applesauce mixture into the baking dishes, sprinkle remaining sugar on top, and bake them in a preheated 375°F (190°C) oven for 15 minutes. Top should be puffed and brown. Serve immediately.

Yield: 6 servings

Each serving contains:

**calories: 171 total fat: 3.5 g saturated fat: 1.1 g cholesterol: 142 mg
sodium: 44 mg carbohydrates: 31.9 g dietary fiber: 0.8 g**

Raspberry Bavarian Pie

An elegant company dessert.

1 pint	fat-free frozen raspberry yogurt	500 mL
12 oz.	frozen raspberries, juice reserved	340 g
1 pkg.	raspberry gelatin	1 pkg.
2	pie shells (not included in totals below)	2

Thaw the frozen yogurt on a plate in the refrigerator for about three hours or until it becomes soft. Thaw the raspberries, reserving the juice. Prepare the gelatin according to the directions on the box, substituting raspberry juice from the thawed raspberries for as much water as possible. Pour into a mixing bowl. Chill the gelatin until it becomes syrupy. Using an electric mixer, whip until double in bulk, fluffy, and thick. Stir in the raspberries and the thawed frozen yogurt. Mix quickly until combined. Pour into pie shells and refrigerate an hour or more.

Yield: 12 servings

Each serving contains:
**calories: 51 total fat: 0.3 g saturated fat: 0 g cholesterol: 0 mg
sodium: 18 mg carbohydrates: 12.1 g dietary fiber: 3.3 g**

Cottage Cheese Pie

Serve with strawberries or other fruit.

¼ C	graham cracker crumbs	310 mL
¼ C	butter or margarine, melted	60 mL
⅛ t	cinnamon (optional)	1 mL
1¾ C	fat-free cottage cheese	435 mL
4 t	cornstarch	20 mL
⅓ C	sugar	80 mL
1 t	vanilla extract	5 mL
1 t	lemon extract	5 mL
2	eggs, separated	2
¼ C	fat-free sour cream	60 mL

Mix together the graham cracker crumbs, melted butter, and cinnamon (if desired) and press onto the sides and bottom of a 9 inch (22 cm) pie plate prepared with nonstick cooking spray. In a mixing bowl, combine the cottage cheese, cornstarch, sugar, extracts, and egg yolks. Beat until smooth. In another bowl, beat the egg whites until stiff peaks form. Fold the egg whites into the cheese mixture. Spoon it carefully into the prepared pie plate. Bake in a preheated 350°F (180°C) oven for 25 minutes. Cool on wire rack. Smooth the sour cream over the top.

Yield: 8 servings

Each serving contains:
**calories: 146 total fat: 2.6 g saturated fat: 0.7 g cholesterol: 58 mg
sodium: 233 mg carbohydrates: 23 g dietary fiber: 0.1 g**

INDEX